Ultrasound: Part 1

Editor

TERESA S. WU

CRITICAL CARE CLINICS

www.criticalcare.theclinics.com

Consulting Editor
RICHARD W. CARLSON

January 2014 • Volume 30 • Number 1

ELSEVIER

1600 John F. Kennedy Boulevard ● Suite 1800 ● Philadelphia, Pennsylvania, 19103-2899

http://www.theclinics.com

CRITICAL CARE CLINICS Volume 30, Number 1
January 2014 ISSN 0749-0704, ISBN-13: 978-0-323-26384-9

Editor: Patrick Manley

Critical Care Clinics (ISSN: 0749-0704) is published quarterly by Elsevier Inc., 360 Park Avenue South, New York, NY 10010-1710. Months of issue are January, April, July, and October. Business and Editorial Offices: 1600 John F. Kennedy Blvd., Suite 1800, Philadelphia, PA 19103-2899. Customer Service Office: 6277 Sea Harbor Drive, Orlando, FL 32887-4800. Periodicals postage paid at New York, NY and additional mailing offices. Subscription prices are $210.00 per year for US individuals, $503.00 per year for US institution, $100.00 per year for US students and residents, $255.00 per year for Canadian individuals, $630.00 per year for Canadian institutions, $300.00 per year for international individuals, $630.00 per year for international institutions and $150.00 per year for Canadian and foreign students/residents. To receive student/resident rate, orders must be accompanied by name of affiliated institution, date of term, and the signature of program/residency coordinator on institution letterhead. Orders will be billed at individual rate until proof of status is received. Foreign air speed delivery is included in all *Clinics* subscription prices. All prices are subject to change without notice. POSTMASTER: Send address changes to *Critical Care Clinics*, Elsevier Periodicals Customer Service, 11830 Westline Industrial Drive, St. Louis, MO 63146. **Customer Service: 1-800-654-2452 (US). From outside of the US, call 1-314-447-8871. Fax: 1-314-447-8029. E-mail: journalscustomerservice-usa@elsevier.com (for print support) or journalsonlinesupport-usa@elsevier.com (for online support).**

Reprints. For copies of 100 or more of articles in this publication, please contact the Commercial Reprints Department, Elsevier Inc., 360 Park Avenue South, New York, NY 10010-1710. Tel.: 212-633-3874; Fax: 212-633-3820; E-mail: reprints@elsevier.com.

Critical Care Clinics is also published in Spanish by Editorial Inter-Medica, Junin 917, 1er A, 1113, Buenos Aires, Argentina.

Critical Care Clinics is covered in *MEDLINE/PubMed (Index Medicus), EMBASE/Excerpta Medica, Current Concepts/Clinical Medicine, ISI/BIOMED,* and *Chemical Abstracts.*

Printed and bound by CPI Group (UK) Ltd, Croydon, CR0 4YY

Transferred to digital print 2012

Contributors

CONSULTING EDITOR

RICHARD W. CARLSON, MD, PhD
Chairman Emeritus, Director, Medical Intensive Care Unit, Department of Medicine, Maricopa Medical Center; Professor, University of Arizona College of Medicine; Professor, Department of Medicine, Mayo Graduate School of Medicine, Phoenix, Arizona

EDITOR

TERESA S. WU, MD, FACEP
Director, Emergency Medicine Ultrasound Program and Fellowship; Co-Director, Simulation Based Training Program and Fellowship; Associate Director, EM Residency Program; Associate Professor, Department of Emergency Medicine, Maricopa Medical Center, University of Arizona, College of Medicine-Phoenix, Phoenix, Arizona

AUTHORS

J. LUIS ENRIQUEZ, MD
Emergency Ultrasound Fellow, Pediatric Emergency Medicine Faculty, Department of Emergency Medicine, Maricopa Medical Center, Phoenix, Arizona

LALEH GHARAHBAGHIAN, MD
Clinical Assistant Professor; Director of Emergency Ultrasound Program and Fellowship, Division of Emergency Medicine, Department of Surgery, Stanford University Medical Center, Stanford, California

VIVETA LOBO, MD
Clinical Instructor, Coordinator of Medical Student and Resident Ultrasound Education, Ultrasound Fellow, Division of Emergency Medicine, Department of Surgery, Stanford University Medical Center, Stanford, California

PHILLIPS PERERA, MD, RDMS
Clinical Associate Professor; Director of Emergency Ultrasound Research; Associate Director of Emergency Ultrasound Program, Division of Emergency Medicine, Department of Surgery, Stanford University Medical Center, Stanford, California

JESSE SHRIKI, DO, MS, RDMS
Director Emergency Ultrasound, Department of Emergency Medicine, Scottsdale Healthcare, Scottsdale, Arizona; Clinical Associate Professor, The University of Arizona, Tucson, Arizona

DANIEL WEINGROW, DO
Assistant Professor; Director of Ultrasound Education, Department of Emergency Medicine, UCLA Olive View/Ronald Reagan Medical Center, Sylmar, California

SARAH R. WILLIAMS, MD
Clinical Associate Professor; Associate Residency Director, Stanford/Kaiser Emergency Medicine Residency Program; Founder and Director Emeritus of Ultrasound Program and Fellowship, Division of Emergency Medicine, Department of Surgery, Stanford University Medical Center, Stanford, California

TERESA S. WU, MD, FACEP
Director, Emergency Medicine Ultrasound Program and Fellowship; Co-Director, Simulation Based Training Program and Fellowship; Associate Director, EM Residency Program; Associate Professor, Department of Emergency Medicine, Maricopa Medical Center, University of Arizona, College of Medicine-Phoenix, Phoenix, Arizona

Contents

Bedside ultrasound has become an important modality for obtaining critical information in the acute care of patients. It is important to understand the physics of ultrasound in order to perform and interpret images at the bedside. The physics of both continuous wave and pulsed wave sound underlies diagnostic ultrasound. The instrumentation, including transducers and image processing, is important in the acquisition of appropriate sonographic images. Understanding how these concepts interplay with each other enables practitioners to obtain the best possible images.

The use of ultrasonography in medical practice has evolved dramatically over the last few decades and will continue to improve as technological advances are incorporated into daily medical practice. Although ultrasound machine size and equipment have evolved, the basic principles and fundamental functions have remained essentially the same. This article reviews the general ultrasound apparatus design, the most common probe types available, and the system controls used to manipulate the images obtained. Becoming familiar with the machine and the controls used for image generation optimizes the scans being performed and enhances the use of ultrasound in patient care.

Focused cardiac echocardiography has become a critical diagnostic tool for both the emergency and critical care physician caring for patients with chest pain, shortness of breath, in a shock state or following trauma to the chest. Bedside echocardiography allows for the immediate diagnosis of pericardial effusion and pericardial tamponade, evaluation of cardiac contractility and volume status, and detection of right ventricular strain seen with a significant pulmonary embolus. The article addresses how to perform focused echocardiography using the standard cardiac windows, how to interpret the acquired images and how to best apply this information clinically at the bedside.

Thoracic ultrasonography (US) has proven to be a valuable tool in the evaluation of the patient with shortness of breath, chest pain, hypoxia, or after chest trauma. Its sensitivity and specificity for detecting disease is higher than that of a chest radiograph, and it can expedite the diagnosis for many emergent conditions. This article describes the technique of each thoracic US application, illustrating both normal and abnormal findings, as well as discussing the relevant literature. Bedside thoracic US has defined imaging benefits in a wide range of thoracic diseases. Furthermore, US guidance has been shown to facilitate thoracic and airway procedures.

This article reviews important literature on the FAST and E-FAST examinations. It also reviews key pitfalls, limitations, and controversies of these examinations. A practical "how-to" guide is presented. Lastly, new frontiers are explored.

Critically ill patients require rapid, accurate assessments and appropriate therapeutic interventions to maximize their chances of recovery. Often the cause of a patient's decompensation is not readily apparent based solely on history and physical examination findings. The Concentrated Overview of Resuscitative Efforts (CORE scan) is a compilation of targeted bedside ultrasound exams that should be performed during the assessment and management of critically ill patients. The CORE scan can be used to help make critical diagnoses and guide resuscitation efforts in patients with undifferentiated deterioration.

CRITICAL CARE CLINICS

DOWNLOAD
Free App!

Review Articles
THE CLINICS

NOW AVAILABLE FOR YOUR iPhone and iPad

Preface

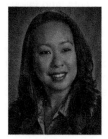

Teresa S. Wu, MD, FACEP
Editor

Over the last few decades, we have witnessed the emergence, acceptance, and utilization of one of the greatest tools in modern medicine. Although the physics of ultrasound was first described in the late 1700s, it wasn't until the late 1980s when ultrasound began to surface as a practical and useful tool in the assessment and management of patients. Pioneers in the field of point-of-care ultrasound faced open opposition and disparagement when the concept of bedside ultrasonography was first introduced, and lack of interdisciplinary collaboration delayed its inevitable implementation into the various realms of medical practice.

We have now entered into an era where ultrasound has become one of the most invaluable tools in imaging and assessing patients. Almost every medical and surgical specialty is using point-of-care ultrasound for procedural guidance, patient assessment, characterization, and diagnosis. Medical students are being introduced to ultrasound in their pre-clinical years, residents from all different specialties are learning how to integrate point-of-care ultrasound into their clinical practice, and fellows are training in advanced ultrasound applications and technologies all over the world.

With its ability to provide real-time, dynamic data in a quick and noninvasive manner at the patient's bedside, it is no wonder that ultrasound has effectively become integrated into all aspects of medicine. The full scope and benefits of point-of-care ultrasonography have grown to such an extent that no single issue of *Critical Care Clinics* can fully address the topic in the detail and manner to which it deserves to be covered. What we hope to do with the two full issues dedicated to ultrasound is to introduce and discuss the most popular and influential ultrasound applications that are currently being employed, and to provide readers with the requisite knowledge and proficiency required to use it in their daily practice.

We are extremely grateful to the many experts who have contributed to the comprehensive and informative articles that are included in the two ultrasound issues of *Critical Care Clinics*, and we have the sincerest appreciation for the members of the editorial board that have worked so hard to bring this publication to fruition. I hope that our overview of point-of-care ultrasonography serves as a launching pad for further reading and research and inspires all that read it to go out and learn how to use ultrasound to help their patients.

Crit Care Clin 30 (2014) ix–x
http://dx.doi.org/10.1016/j.ccc.2013.10.001

This edition of *Critical Care Clinics* is dedicated to all of my mentors and educators who have instilled in me the knowledge, passion, and dedication to advance medical education and improve patient care and to all of my students, residents, and fellows, who continue to challenge and inspire me with their eagerness to learn and willingness to be taught. To Dr Richard Carlson who had the insight and foresight to support global, multi-disciplinary education about point-of-care ultrasound. To my mother, Phyllis Wu, whose sacrifices and guidance have enabled me to pursue my dreams and be the educator and physician I am today. And, finally, to my husband, Thomas Pearson, and my wonderful children, Kai and Kenna, whose love, laughter, and support have made all things possible.

Teresa S. Wu, MD, FACEP
Department of Emergency Medicine
Maricopa Medical Center
University of Arizona
College of Medicine–Phoenix
2601 East Roosevelt Street
Phoenix, AZ 85008, USA

E-mail address:
teresawumd@gmail.com

Ultrasound Physics

Jesse Shriki, DO, MS, RDMS[a,b]

KEYWORDS

- Ultrasound physics • Frequency • Period • Transducer • Instrumentation
- Doppler shift

KEY POINTS

- This article introduces the physics essential for understanding diagnostic medical ultrasound.
- This article discusses the differences between continuous wave and pulsed wave ultrasound.
- The basics of ultrasound instrumentation, such as transducers and display modes, are explained.
- Ultrasound techniques, such as Doppler imaging, are introduced.
- An understanding of key concepts, such as resolution and artifact, are discussed.

INTRODUCTION

Point-of-care emergency ultrasound has become the modern-day physician's stethoscope equivalent. The concepts fundamental to ultrasound physics are critical in both understanding point-of-care ultrasound and obtaining the best possible images. Without knowledge of how the ultrasound system interprets and acquires sound waves, understanding the perceived anatomy can be difficult at best. Knowing how the images are created can help practitioners determine if an image produced is an accurate depiction of the anatomy or if artifacts are confounding (or contributing) to the acquired images.

BASIC SOUND

In order to understand diagnostic ultrasound, sound should be thought of as more than just the familiar sense of hearing. Rather, sound should be thought of as the interaction of energy and matter. In contradistinction to electromagnetic energy, sound is mechanical energy transmitted by pressure waves in a medium,[1] which means that sound exists in the form of particles moving in a medium. A sound source, such as a tuning fork, acts like a piston pushing waves of vibration longitudinally through

The author listed has identified no professional or financial affiliations.
[a] Department of Emergency Medicine, Scottsdale Emergency Associates, 7400 E Osborn Avenue, Scottsdale, AZ 85251, USA; [b] The University of Arizona, Tucson, AZ 85721, USA
E-mail address: Shrikido@gmail.com

tissue. The sound wave produced has areas of high pressure (or high density) and low pressure (or low density). The high-pressure areas (compression) are where the sound waves are compressed together and the low-pressure areas (rarefaction) are where the sound waves are spaced apart (**Fig. 1**).

Sound particles should be thought of as elements of transverse and longitudinal waveforms moving in a medium. In diagnostic ultrasound, the media can be air, blood, or soft tissue. In the absence of media (ie, a vacuum), sound cannot propagate. In a transverse wave, displacement of the medium is perpendicular to the direction of propagation of the wave, as in a ripple on a pond. In longitudinal waves, the displacement of the medium is parallel to the propagation of the wave, moving like a Slinky or caterpillar back and forth (**Fig. 2**). Only longitudinal waves effectively traverse distances and, therefore, only longitudinal waves are important in diagnostic ultrasound.

SOUND SOURCE

The production of sound requires an oscillating or vibrating source. A tuning fork is a good example of how sound is produced by oscillation and vibration (see **Fig. 1**). When a tuning fork vibrates, it moves adjacent air molecules causing them, in turn, to vibrate. Sound spreads throughout the medium, air, as a wave in all directions.

In the ultrasound system, the sound source is a piezoelectric crystal, such as quartz. Modern transducers typically use a lead zirconate titanate (PZT) amalgam. The piezoelectric effect allows for these crystals to vibrate when an electrical voltage is applied across it and subsequently creates sound waves. Conversely, piezoelectric crystals also can convert sound waves back into electrical energy so that the sound waves can be converted into data that can be processed into anatomic images.

WAVES

A single-frequency sound wave is commonly conceptualized as a single sine wave causing alternating pressure variations in the air (**Fig. 4**). Ultrasound waves are rarely, however, waves of a single frequency and are generally made up of multiple frequencies. Accordingly, these waves can interfere with each other either constructively or destructively (**Fig. 3**).[1]

ACOUSTIC PARAMETER AND VARIABLES

To understand the basic physics of ultrasound, acoustic parameters and acoustic variables must be defined; they are the basis of describing waves. In physics nomenclature,

Longitudinal Wave

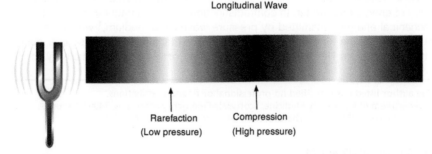

Rarefaction   Compression
(Low pressure)   (High pressure)

Fig. 1. The tuning fork acts like a piston, creating sound waves of areas of high pressure (represented by the *black areas*) and low pressure (represented by *white areas*).

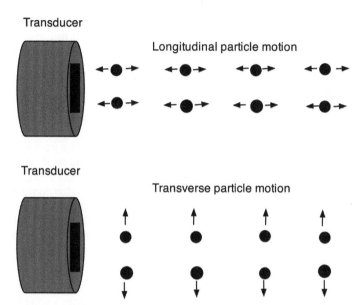

Transducer

Longitudinal particle motion

Transducer

Transverse particle motion

Fig. 2. Particle wave motion. The top shows a transducer with longitudinal particle waves. The bottom shows transverse particle motion. Only longitudinal waves can produce ultrasound waves that provide useful diagnostic information.

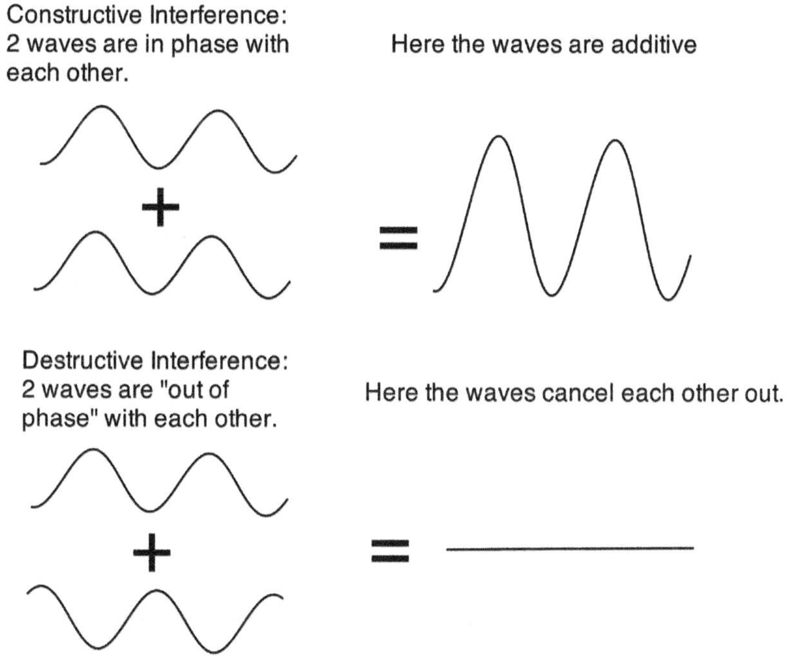

Constructive Interference: 2 waves are in phase with each other.

Here the waves are additive

Destructive Interference: 2 waves are "out of phase" with each other.

Here the waves cancel each other out.

Fig. 3. Waves of varying frequencies can increase (*top*) or decrease (*bottom*) the resultant wave as in constructive interference or destructive interference, respectively.

sound waves are defined by acoustic variables and characterized by acoustic parameters. Acoustic variables are pressure, density, and distance and help define a sound wave. Once the sound wave is defined, it can be described by its frequency, amplitude, power, intensity, wavelength, and propagation speed.

PERIOD AND FREQUENCY

The most well-known acoustic variables are period and frequency. Period is the time to complete a single cycle. It can also be stated as the time from the start of 1 cycle to the start of the next cycle (see **Fig. 4**). In ultrasound, period is the time from the start of 1 peak, including 1 valley, to the next peak. Typical values in diagnostic ultrasound for period are expressed in microseconds. Frequency is the number of events that occur in a particular time frame. In ultrasound, the frequency of a wave is the number of cycles that occur in 1 second. Typical frequencies in diagnostic ultrasound are expressed in megahertz. Ultrasound transducer frequencies vary from 1 MHz to 15 MHz. Given this inverse relationship, period and frequency are the reciprocal of each other.[1]

WAVELENGTH

The distance between 1 peak and the next represents 1 cycle; it is the distance between 2 similar points on corresponding waves and represents 1 wavelength. It is a simple but important concept to understand that wavelength is a distance, whereas period is a time (see **Fig. 4**). Typical diagnostic ultrasound wavelengths are in the millimeter range. Wavelength (λ) and frequency (f) are also inversely related to one another,

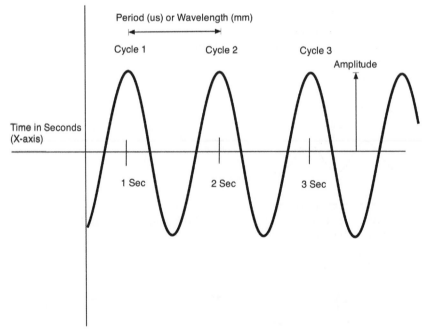

Fig. 4. Graphic representation of a single-frequency sound wave with labeled period and amplitude. The frequency of this wave is 3 cycles per second, or 3 Hz. Note that period and wavelength are similar terms; period represents time and wavelength represents distance. The amplitude is the value of the wave from the zero of the Y axis to the top of the wave.

and their product is the speed (v) of sound in a medium (**Fig. 5**). Sound is presumed to travel at 1540 m/s in soft tissue, which is approximately 1 mile per second. Therefore, sound of a 1-MHz frequency has a wavelength of 1.54 mm.

$$v = fx\lambda$$

Fig. 5. Speed of sound (v) is the product of frequency (f) and wavelength (λ).

PARAMETERS OF MAGNITUDE

So far, the time parameters in which a wave occurs have been described. The next 3 parameters describe the magnitude and strength (or "bigness") of the sound wave. These parameters are amplitude, power, and intensity. In conjunction with acoustic variables, these parameters are important in describing how the waves interact with the medium. Additionally, these parameters build on each other and are mathematically related to each other.

Amplitude is the size of the wave. Graphically, it is the difference between the maximum value and the average value of the wave. Amplitude is the strength of the wave measured from the zero line to the top of the wave (see **Fig. 4**). Power is the next parameter and is defined as the energy (joules) generated per unit of time. It can also be thought of as the rate of at which work is performed. Power is expressed in watts. Output of a light bulb or a stereo is also expressed in watts and can be thought of as another example of power. In diagnostic ultrasound, a sonographer can adjust output power. By increasing the voltage to the crystal, the force of vibration is increased. Stronger sound waves are transmitted into the body and, subsequently, make an image brighter (**Fig. 6**).

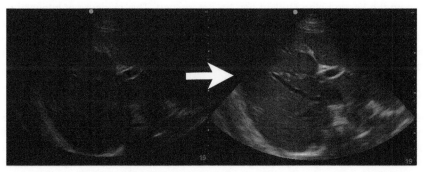

Fig. 6. Increasing the output power allows for a change in brightness to the overall image. It increases the strength of both the strong and weak reflectors making the entire image brighter (*arrow* denotes before and after gain change).

Lastly and, most importantly, is intensity, which has a direct affect on the bioeffects of ultrasound on human tissue. Intensity is defined as the concentration of the energy in the cross-section of the sound beam. It is calculated as the power divided by the cross-sectional area of the sound wave (**Fig. 7**).

$$Intensity(I) = \frac{Power[Watts]}{Area[cm^2]}$$

Fig. 7. Intensity equation as it relates the power to the area. Intensity is the concentration of energy in a beam.

Intensity is directly related to power. Moreover, both intensity and power are related through the amplitude. For the purposes of this review, both power and intensity are directly proportional to the square of the amplitude (**Fig. 8**).

$$Intensity \propto Amplitude^2$$

$$Power \propto Amplitude^2$$

Fig. 8. The relationship of intensity and power to amplitude. Notice that mathematically power and intensity are proportional to each other.

For example, if the amplitude of the wave is tripled, then the power and the intensity are both increased 9-fold. The magnitude parameters can all be changed by a sonographer during a bedside scan.[2]

ROLE OF INTENSITY

An important consideration is that intensity is not uniform across any one particular sound wave. Just as a stereo does not supply the same quality of sound in every single point in a room, the intensity of a sound wave can vary across any given space. Intensities can thus be measured differently for each sound beam. Intensity may be measure at its highest (peak) intensity or overall intensity. Intensity may also be measured over time. For example, longer measurement times change the exposure to the tissue. Intensity of the beam measured over time is called temporal variation and over space is called spatial variation.

Although intensity can be measured temporally or spatially, one specific measurement of intensity should be discussed. By measuring the peak spatial and average time intensity, or spatial peak–temporal average (SPTA), the effect of the sound wave on the tissue being studied can be determined. This measure of intensity can be thought of as the peak intensity that the tissues absorb during medical ultrasound. When determining the effect of ultrasound on biologic tissue, the SPTA is what is measured and used for a marker of harm.[3] For now, remember that with any type of energy, some is absorbed and dissipated as heat.

PROPAGATION SPEED

The last of the acoustic parameters is propagation speed, which is defined as the distance that a sound wave travels through a medium in 1 second. In general, sound travels fastest in solids, slower in liquids, and slowest in gases. In the human body, the speed of sound varies. It can range anywhere from 500 m/s to 4000 m/s, depending on the tissue. On average, the propagation speed of soft tissue is approximately 1540 m/s. By comparison, lung propagation speed is 500 m/s, and bone propagation speed is 3500 m/s. Propagation speed depends solely on the medium. There are certain characteristics of a medium that affect propagation speed. Those characteristics are stiffness and density. Propagation speed is proportional to stiffness and inversely proportional to density. A medium with increased stiffness (ie, bone) has an increased propagation speed. A medium with increased density has a slower speed. For example, because bone is stiff and not dense, it has the fastest propagation speed. Conversely, lung tissue, because it is compressible (not stiff) and dense has the slowest speed (**Fig. 9**).[1]

ATTENUATION

The concept of attenuation is a major contributor to the quality of images. Attenuation is the weakening of sound as it travels longer distances (ie, through deeper tissue).

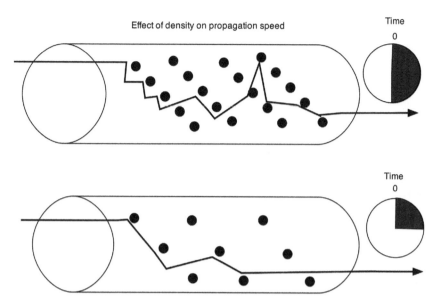

Fig. 9. The effect of density on propagation speed. The arrow represents a sound wave. The numbers of dots represent varying density. The top is an example of a material with an increased density causing slower propagation speed (more objects to maneuver). The bottom is an example of a low-density material with a fast propagation speed.

Additionally, higher frequencies weaken more than lower frequencies. Therefore, deeper imaging and higher frequencies attenuate the most, whereas shallow imaging and lower frequencies attenuate the least. Consequently, the strength parameters of amplitude, power, and intensity all decrease as a function of depth and frequency, highlighting a major concept: changing the depth actually changes the brightness of the image. To obtain the best images possible, the shallowest depth should be used (**Fig. 10**).

The unit of attenuation is the decibel. The decibel is not an absolute measure of intensity but rather a relative measure. The decibel is a logarithmic scale comparing

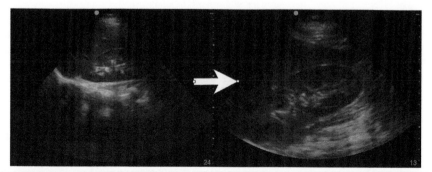

Fig. 10. Changing imaging depth changes the attenuation. Imaging of Morison pouch. Deeper imaging results in more attenuation. Notice here the lack of detail of the kidney in the left panel. The left panel is also brighter because of reflection from the diaphragm (*arrow* denotes before and after depth change).

2 intensities. This scale is similar to that of pH, such that decibels change exponentially rather than arithmetically. As a rule of thumb, a 10-dB change in intensity corresponds to a 10-fold change. Hence, a change of 50 dB implies a 100,000-fold change (10^5).

EFFECT OF TISSUE

Intrinsic to different types of tissue (liver, muscle, fat, and so forth) is that each has its own effect on attenuation, called the tissue's attenuation coefficient. The attenuation coefficient is measured in decibels per centimeter. In soft tissue, the attenuation coefficient is approximately half the transducer frequency or approximately 0.5 dB/cm/MHz.[4,5] Thus, an 8-MHz transducer in soft tissue has an attenuation coefficient of 4 dB/cm. If the object of interest were 8 cm away, then the total attenuation is 32 dB ($8 \times 4 = 32$), a 1000-fold change.

Some specific media deserve special mention. In water, there is no noticeable attenuation of frequencies of 10 MHz or less, making it an excellent acoustic window. Muscle tissue, due to its directional fiber bundles, can vary in the amount of attenuation depending on the orientation of the sound beams to the fibers. Sound attenuation increases twice as much when it travels perpendicular to the muscle fibers as opposed to its attenuation parallel to its fibers.[2] This directional dependence of the fibers on the attenuation is known as anisotropy. It is the reason that occasionally muscle fibers appear dark and may be mistaken for vascular structures (**Fig. 11**).

REFLECTION

There are 3 major causes of attenuation; they are reflection, scatter, and absorption. Reflection is the amount of sound returned to the sound source or transducer. Transmission is the amount of sound that passes through the tissue. Transmission is useless in diagnostic medical ultrasound where image production relies on reflection back to the probe. Reflection occurs due to the interaction of sound at an interface of 2 media. The amount of echoes returning to the sound source depends on how much reflection occurs. Different types of reflectors cause different amounts of reflection. Reflectors that have a smooth surface (specular reflectors) cause organized sound to be reflected back to the transducer. Reflectors that have a rough surface (diffuse reflectors) cause scattered sound to be reflected, some of which goes back to the transducer. A particular type of scatter occurs when a reflectors' surface is

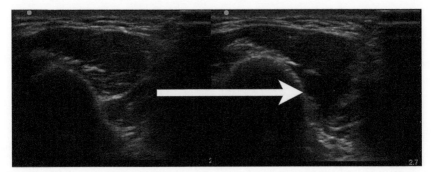

Fig. 11. Ultrasound of muscle fibers in the forearm. The fibers display anisotropy. Note the brightness of the muscle fibers on the left panel. The right panel contains the exact same image changing only the incident angle of the probe on the forearm. Consequently the muscle bundles appear hypoechoic.

much smaller than the beam's wavelength, called Rayleigh scattering, the same type of organized scatter that occurs when a stone causes ripples in a pond. In the body, red blood cells display Rayleigh scattering (**Fig. 12**).[2]

The angle of incidence of sound also greatly affects the reflection. The physics of perpendicular incidence is simpler than that of oblique incidence. The amount of reflections that occur with perpendicular incidence is determined solely by a property intrinsic to each tissue, called the acoustic impedance. The acoustic impedance of a medium affects the strength of the reflected sound. At a perpendicular incidence, the difference between the impedance of 2 media is the only factor that effects reflection. If the difference in impedance between 2 media's interface is too great, then sound waves are completely reflected.[2] The percent of sound reflected may be calculated as a ratio of the impedance of the different media (**Fig. 13**). As an example, air has infinitesimally low impedance in comparison to tissue (eg, muscle).[1] When sound waves come in contact with air, the sound waves almost completely reflect back; thus, no transmission can be seen when there is air at the interface.[1]

In contradistinction to perpendicular incidence, oblique incidence sound causes the reflected beam to travel off at an angle. The physics of reflection with oblique incidence is much more complicated. The incident angle at which the sound strikes the

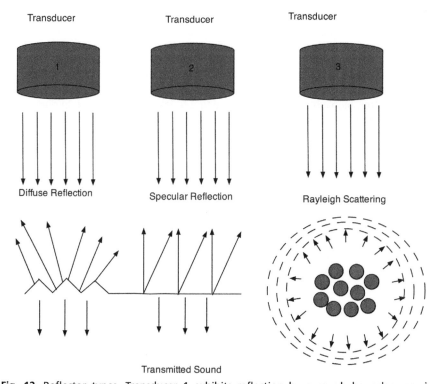

Fig. 12. Reflector types. Transducer 1 exhibits reflection by a rough boundary causing diffuse scatter, some of which go back to the transducer. Transducer 2 exhibits reflection by a smooth (specular) boundary causing organized reflection, much of which goes back to the transducer. Transducer 3 exhibits Rayleigh scattering. Red cells scatter sound concentrically in all directions because they are much smaller than the wavelength of diagnostic ultrasound.

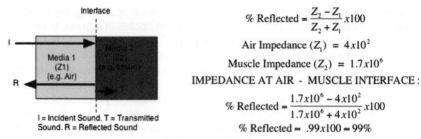

$$\% \text{ Reflected} = \frac{Z_2 - Z_1}{Z_2 + Z_1} x100$$

Air Impedance (Z_1) = $4x10^2$

Muscle Impedance (Z_2) = $1.7x10^6$

IMPEDANCE AT AIR - MUSCLE INTERFACE:

$$\% \text{ Reflected} = \frac{1.7x10^6 - 4x10^2}{1.7x10^6 + 4x10^2} x100$$

$\% \text{ Reflected} \approx .99x100 \approx 99\%$

I = Incident Sound. T = Transmitted
Sound. R = Reflected Sound

Fig. 13. Effect of impedance (Z) on reflection. Calculation of the percent of reflected sound with an air interface. It can be seen that because air has such smaller impedance, any air-tissue (here, muscle tissue) interface has 99% reflection.

reflector equals the reflected angle at which the sound leaves that reflector, yielding reflection but with a bend. Reflection with a bend is the definition of refraction. Refraction can become a clinically important artifact. Refraction is greatest at bone and soft tissue interfaces (**Fig. 14**).

SCATTER

Scatter is the redirection of sound in many directions (see **Fig. 12**). Sound scatters when the tissue interface is smaller than the wavelength of the sound waves it receives. Lung tissue scatters sound due to the air-filled alveoli. In general, the amount of scatter is directly proportional to frequency. So, higher-frequency sound scatters more than lower-frequency sound. Frequency increases exponentially with increased Rayleigh scatter, highlighting another critical fact to learn from physics. In diagnostic ultrasound, the goal is to use the highest frequency possible to provide the best images, but this comes with the cost of increased scatter.

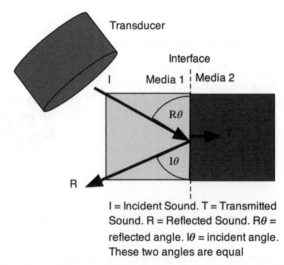

I = Incident Sound. T = Transmitted
Sound. R = Reflected Sound. Rθ =
reflected angle. Iθ = incident angle.
These two angles are equal

Fig. 14. Refraction. The incident angle at which the sound strikes the reflector equals the reflected angle at which the sound leaves that reflector.

Scatter is the reason different echogenic structures can be seen within a particular tissue. For example, during a scan, a hemangioma can be seen in the liver parenchyma due to different levels of scattering within the liver tissue (**Fig. 15**). The hyperechoic hemangioma produces more scattering than the surrounding liver parenchyma. Similarly, hypoechoic areas, like cysts, have a scattering level lower than in the surrounding tissue.[2]

ABSORPTION

The final cause of attenuation is absorption. Absorption occurs when acoustic energy is converted into heat, which is also a major cause of attenuation.[4] The amount of absorption increases as both transducer frequency and scanning depth increase. The greater the absorption, the more heat is generated. Under normal diagnostic scanning conditions, however, the amount of heat produced is too small to cause any measurable temperature changes.[1,3]

PULSED SOUND

Thus far, single-frequency sound waves as they travel through time have been described. Sound is commonly depicted as a single sinusoidal (or continuous) wave in time (see **Fig. 4**). Continuous wave sound cannot, however, create anatomic images. Diagnostic ultrasound uses short pulses of sound to create anatomic images. Therefore, parameters of pulse sound in addition to continuous sound must be described.

A pulse is collections of cycles that travel together.[2] Transducers emit pulses of sound waves. Each transducer emits a pulse with a set duration, called the pulse duration. Pulse duration is the time from the start of a pulse to the end of pulse. It can also be described as the transmit time. In-between pulses, the transducer is listening for the return of these pulses after they are reflected back. The time in-between pulses is the receive time. In diagnostic ultrasound, the ideal transducer uses pulses of a very short duration. Shorter pulses can discriminate between smaller objects (resolution).[2] Spatial pulse length is the length of each pulse. Because each transducer pulse is identical to the next, the pulses are repetitions of each other. The pulse repetition

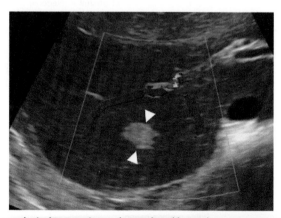

Fig. 15. The hyperechoic hemangioma (*arrowheads*) produces more scattering than the surrounding liver parenchyma. Similarly, hypoechoic areas, like cysts, have a scattering level lower than in the surrounding tissue. (*Data from* Edelman SK. Understanding ultrasound physics. ESP; 2005.)

period (PRP) is defined as the time from the start of 1 pulse to the start of the next pulse. It includes 1 transmit time plus 1 receive time. The pulse repetition frequency (PRF) is the number of pulses in 1 second. Similar to continuous wave, in pulsed wave, period (PRP) and frequency (PRF) are reciprocals of each other (**Fig. 16**).

Pulsed ultrasound can be thought of similarly to boxcars on a train (**Fig. 17**).[2] PRP and PRF are both related to the imaging depth. The pulses are all of the same duration, so with deeper imaging, only the receive time, or "listening" time, in-between pulses changes. Increasing PRP equals increasing listening time and corresponds to deeper imaging because deeper sound waves have to travel further and the sound waves take longer to return, requiring longer listening times. Accordingly, PRF is inversely proportional to imaging depth. More cycles means shorter listening time (**Fig. 18**).[2]

INSTRUMENTATION

In addition to understanding the physics of sound, basic instrumentation that creates and interprets sound must be understood. Pulsed wave ultrasound creates 2-D images using the characteristics of the sound received. The transducer is only one part of that system. The specific design and function of the various components of a real-time imaging system are complex and sophisticated; however, all systems share some basic components, including the master synchronizer, the transducer, the pulser, the receiver, the storage device, and display. Although some of these components are self-explanatory, the roles of some of these components are discussed briefly.

TRANSDUCER

The transducer is the most recognizable part of the system. At its most basic function, a transducer converts electrical energy into acoustic energy and, conversely, converts acoustic energy into electrical energy during receive times. The transducer can be

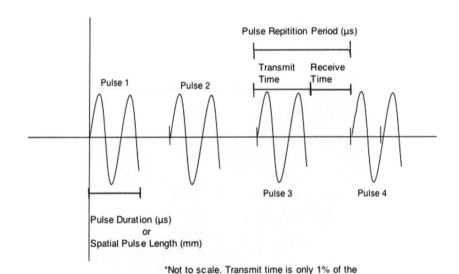

Fig. 16. Parameters of pulsed sound. The PRP is the time from the start of 1 pulse to the start of the next (Transmit Time + Receive Time). Spatial pulse length is the length of each pulse. PRF is the number of pulses per second.

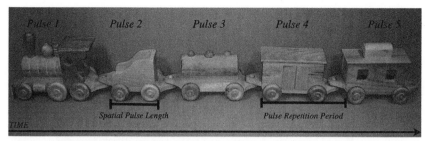

Fig. 17. Parameters of pulsed sound–boxcar analogy. Spatial pulse length is the length of each boxcar. The PRP is the time from the start of 1 boxcar to the start of the next (transmit plus receive time). PRF is the number of boxcars (here, 5) that pass in 1 second.

thought of as both a microphone and a speaker. Although actual transducers themselves are complicated, they can be broken down into simplified components. As stated previously, transducers contain piezoelectric crystals that allow the conversion of sound into energy. PZT is the active element of the crystals. When a voltage is applied across this active element, it vibrates to create sound waves. Although these crystals can be brittle and rather fragile, modern transducers combine a transducer element with an epoxy resin to make a composite material. Transducers typically contain arrays or sets of multiple active elements.

In addition to the active element, transducers have 6 other components; they are the case, the electrical shield, the insulator, the wire, the matching layer, and the damping element (**Fig. 19**).

The case protects the internal components and insulates the elements so that the applied voltage goes only to the active element and not to the patient or sonographer. For this reason, a cracked transducer case should never be used given the potential to

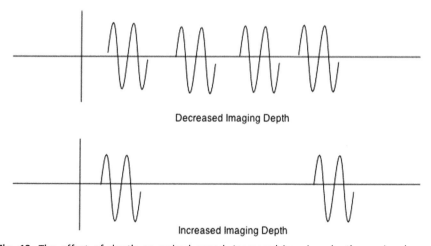

Decreased Imaging Depth

Increased Imaging Depth

Fig. 18. The effect of depth on pulsed sound. Increased imaging depth requires longer pauses between pulses because each pulse takes longer to return. The top represents shallow imaging. It has more cycles (higher PRF) and shorter "listening" times (smaller PRP). The bottom represents deeper imaging. It has fewer cycles (lower PRF) and longer listening times (larger PRP). Note the spatial pulse length and pulse duration do not change.

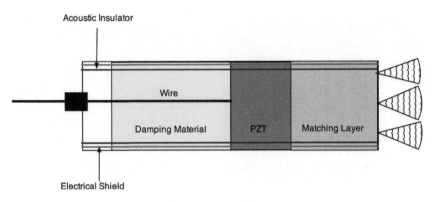

Acoustic Insulator

Wire

Damping Material   PZT   Matching Layer

Electrical Shield

Schematic of a Transducer

Fig. 19. The components of a typical transducer used in diagnostic ultrasound.

electrocute the patient or sonographer. The case is also lined with an electrical shield that prevents ambient electrical noise from causing interference. In addition, there is an acoustic insulator that prevents vibrations in the case from inducing an electrical voltage. A wire provides electrical connection between the crystal and the system. This wire carries the voltage that excites the crystal to its appropriate frequency. The final 2 components are the matching layer and the backing material, which sandwich the crystal. The matching layer is specifically positioned in front of the crystal. It increases the efficiency of sound energy transfer between the element and body. It is a stepping-stone of sorts for sound to traverse the junction between the crystal and body. The impedance of the matching layer is designed to be midway between PZT and skin. As discussed previously, if the sound beam travels from the crystal to the skin directly, much of the sound waves would be reflected due to the large difference in impedance. The lowered impedance of the matching layer is how reflections are decreased at the crystal-skin boundary. Ultrasound gel functions similarly to cause a stepwise decrease in impedance.

A damping material is attached to the opposite side of the crystal. The damping material assists in turning the pulsed waves of sound into short bursts. As stated previously, short pulses create more accurate images. The damping element restricts the deformation of the crystal, thereby resulting in pulses of short duration. In addition, the damping material reduces vibration during reception. Most transducers are capable of producing both continuous wave sound and pulsed wave sound by activating only 1 or multiple elements in the array, respectively.[2]

MASTER SYNCHRONIZER

The accurate acquisition and display of sonographic information is dependent on the interaction of physical and electrical phenomena that occur in fractions of a second. Electrical pulses are sent to multiple elements in a transducer array. Processing these signals and keeping track of all these functions are the jobs of the master synchronizer.[2]

PULSER

To generate ultrasound waves, the transducer crystal needs to vibrate. The pulser causes the crystal to do this by supplying a voltage across the active element. A pulser consists of a clock and a voltage generator. The voltage generator delivers a short, high-amplitude electrical voltage, typically in the range of 150 V to 900 V, and lasts for as little as 1 μs to 2 μs. In more complex systems, a sonographer can increase the output by increasing the voltage. The clock simply controls the timing of the electrical pulses.[1]

RECEIVER

Sound waves returning to the transducer are converted into electrical impulses by the piezoelectric crystal. The returned electrical impulses are raw signals that need to be refined into data that can be easily interpreted. The receiver functions to amplify and clean the signal of the retuned impulses. It does this by performing 5 functions: amplification, compensation, compression, demodulation, and rejection. Although a complete discussion of the receiver functions is beyond the scope of this article, an introduction to these terms is important. These functions can be adjusted during a scan and are basic functions of the ultrasound. Amplification, also called receiver gain, amplifies all the signals equally to increase brightness of the entire image (see **Fig. 6**). Compensation functions to make all echoes from similar reflectors appear identical regardless of the depth. Stated alternatively, it is the ability to make deeper structures brighter, known as time gain compensation (TGC). TGC compensates for absorption because increased gain can be applied specifically to the deeper signals. The TGC knobs appear similar to an equalizer on a radio and are adjustable with depth (**Fig. 20**).[2]

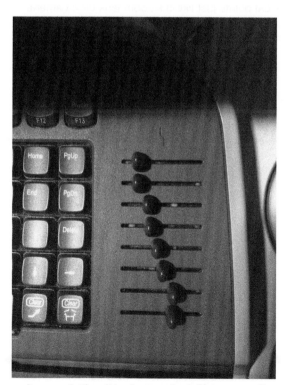

Fig. 20. TGC on an ultrasound. The slider buttons look like an equalizer on a stereo. The gain can be varied with depth. Note here that the gain is increased toward the bottom.

The compression receiver function reduces the total number of signals so that the echo information can be displayed as a 2-D gray-scale image. Demodulation in its simplest form eliminates or corrects for any negative voltages and makes a signal suitable to be seen on a display. Finally, rejection allows for the display of low-level echoes only when they are clinically meaningful, eliminating low-level noise in the desired images.[2]

ANATOMY OF A SOUND BEAM

When a sound wave leaves the transducer, it travels as a beam in a similar fashion to the way a beam of light leaves a flashlight. Initially, the beam width is exactly the same diameter as the transducer, called the aperture, as in photography. The beam progressively narrows like an hourglass until it reaches its smallest diameter and then widens again (**Fig. 21**). The beam is divided into 3 areas: near field, focal point, and far field. The region from the transducer to the midpoint is called the near field. In this area, the beam gradually narrows. The midpoint of the beam, where it is at its narrowest, is the focal point. From the focal point on, the beam widens in the area of the far field. Just like eyes have a distance that is the sharpest for vision, the focal point of the transducer beam produces the sharpest images. Areas arising from the focal zone are more accurate than those from other depths.

When a diagnostic ultrasound is performed, the depth should be adjusted so that the target organ is imaged at the focal zone. Eyes have only one focal point and corrective lenses are needed when that changes with age. Lenses, however, can have adjustable focal points just like the zoom lens on a camera. Some transducers also have adjustable focal points. Transducers that have an adjustable focus are called phased-array transducers.[1]

RESOLUTION

With an understanding of the basics, the property of resolution can be discussed. Resolution is the ability to image accurately. As the name states, it is the measure of how well sound waves can resolve 2 objects that are spatially close to each other. Like a golf score, a lower resolution is preferred. A 2-mm resolution is able to distinguish

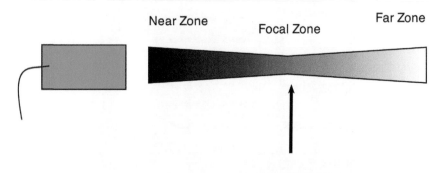

Fig. 21. The anatomy of a sound beam. The transducer (*blue*) is on the left. The near field (near zone) is closest to the transducer. The far field (far zone) is furthest. The narrowest point of the beam is the focal point. The beam diameter at the beginning of the near zone is the same diameter as the transducer lens.

objects better than a 4-mm resolution. In addition to distance, resolution may be defined as separating objects in space (spatial), time (temporal), or shades of gray (contrast).

Spatial resolution is further categorized as axial (parallel to the beam) or lateral (perpendicular to the beam) (**Fig. 22**).

Axial resolution distinguishes structures along the beam's main axis. Shorter pulses create more accurate images. It is known that short pulses have a small wavelength (small spatial pulse length) and short pulse duration. Therefore, higher frequencies (ie, the reciprocal of wavelength) have better resolution (**Fig. 23**). Pulse duration can only be changed by manufacturing properties of the transducer (eg, better damping material).[1] Lateral resolution is the minimum distance that 2 structures are separated when they are side-to-side or perpendicular to the beam. Lateral resolution is best at the narrowest part of the beam and worsens as it moves further away from this focal point (**Fig. 24**). In general, axial resolution is better than lateral resolution because ultrasound pulses are shorter than they are wide.[2]

Temporal resolution is the time it takes to create an image. It is measured by how many frames per second can be created (frame rate), analogous to creating either a good movie or a good photograph. There is a balance between how detailed each image is versus how well the movie flows between frames. Detailed images require a long time to make each frame, thus slow down the movie. Time to create 1 frame, therefore, is inversely related to the frame rate.[2] In diagnostic ultrasound, a shallow image takes less time to create because the beams travel a shorter distance, allowing for a faster frame rate and improved temporal resolution. Temporal resolution is important in scanning moving objects, such as an actively beating heart, and is why a smaller phased-array transducer is used for cardiac imaging. Stationary objects, like the liver

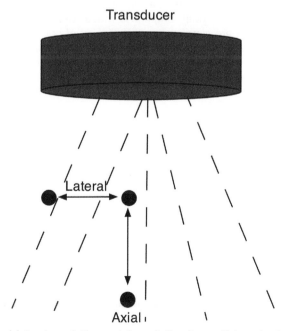

Fig. 22. Axial and lateral resolution: axial resolution is parallel to the beam and lateral resolution is perpendicular to the beam.

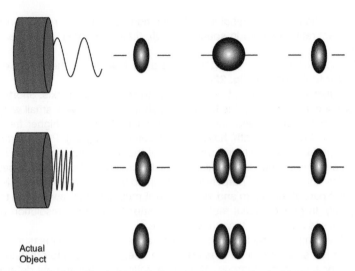

Actual
Object

Fig. 23. Axial resolution. The bottom dots represent the actual objects in space. The top transducer has longer pulse. The lower transducer has a shorter pulse. Shorter pulses can resolve images that are closer together.

and kidney, require less temporal resolution and can be scanned with more detail using a larger 60-mm curvilinear transducer.

DISPLAY MODES

Once the information is gathered, the data can be displayed. There are 3 main display modes: amplitude mode (A-mode), brightness mode (B-mode), and motion mode (M-mode). These modes are simply a graphic display of collected information and comparison of 2 parameters. A-mode is used to measure distance by displaying the amplitude of the wave versus time (ie, depth) for the return of that pulse. Because this mode allows for precise measurements, it was used in ophthalmology for ocular measurements (**Fig. 25**). Its use is limited because A-mode only presents echo data from a single beam.[1]

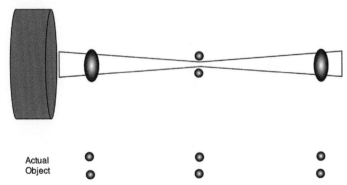

Actual
Object

Fig. 24. Lateral resolution. The bottom dots represent the actual objects in space. The sound beam narrows until the focal point and then widen again. It is in this narrowest part of the beam that the transducer can most accurately resolve images.

A- mode Ultrasound

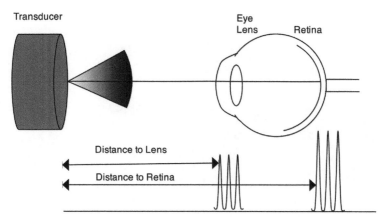

Fig. 25. A-mode: the measured spectrum is a graph of amplitude versus time. The time for a pulse to come back is proportional to the distance.

In B-mode (**Fig. 26**), the varying amplitudes are converted into dots of varying intensity used to generate anatomic images with the depth still proportional to the time of flight of the pulse. Weaker reflections appear as darker gray dots whereas stronger reflections appear as brighter white dots.[2]

Lastly, in M-mode, movement of tissue is displayed. Stationary reflectors are traced out as straight lines, whereas moving reflectors are traced out as sinusoidal lines (**Fig. 27**).

ARTIFACTS

All this information can be used to understand the interpretation of ultrasound images. The physics and instrumentation of ultrasound allow conceptualizing not only how images are formed but also how artifacts are generated. One key difference in ultrasound, as opposed to radiograph, is the presence and utilization of artifacts. In its broadest sense, an artifact is an error in imaging. In ultrasound, however, these artifacts allow obtaining key information about the structures discussed.

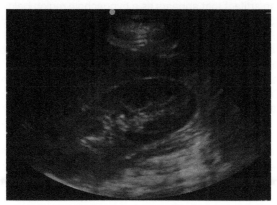

Fig. 26. B-mode: anatomic images are created by displaying reflectors as a function distance from the transducer and intensity of the tissue reflectors.

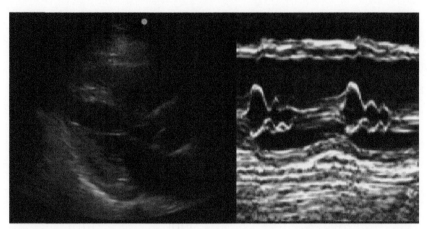

Fig. 27. M-mode: the left panel is a standard B-mode picture. The right panel shows an M-mode tracing of the mitral valve overt time.

Artifacts are made up of reflections that do not occur anatomically and result from a violation of basic assumptions of an imaging system. Six assumptions are incorporated into the design of every ultrasound system. Artifacts occur when these assumptions are not true. These assumptions are

1. Sound travels in a straight line.
2. Sound travels directly to a reflector and back.
3. Sound travels in soft tissue at exactly 1540 m/s.
4. Reflections arise only from structures in the beam's main axis.
5. The imaging plane is very thin.
6. The strength of the reflection is related to the characteristics of the tissue.

Some of the key artifacts seen in diagnostic ultrasound are discussed. The first artifact seen regularly is reverberation artifact (**Fig. 28**). Reverberations appear on the display as multiple equally spaced echoes and are caused by sound bouncing between 2 strong reflectors. The first and second reflections closest to the transducer are real but the remaining do not correspond to true anatomy. Comet tail artifact is a type of reverberation artifact that is typically seen in thoracic ultrasound.

Shadowing is an artifact that appears as a hypoechoic region below a strong attenuating medium. Shadows appear when the attenuation is higher in the tissue above the shadow than in the surrounding tissue. Shadowing is not related to the speed of sound in a medium. Shadowing can confirm the presence of anatomic structures, such as a gallstone (**Fig. 29**).

Edge artifact is a type of shadowing that appears as a hypoechoic region extending along the edge of a curved reflector. Here the sound beam refracts at the edge of a curved reflector and decreases the intensity. Edge artifact can be seen along a normal gallbladder wall (**Fig. 30**) and can be mistaken for the acoustic shadow seen with gallstones.

Lastly, mirror artifact is created when sound reflects off a strong reflector. It is redirected toward a second structure. This redirection causes a replica or a second copy of the structure to appear on the image. This artifact occurs because the system presumes sound to travel in a straight line. Artifact is typically visualized deeper than the real structure. The presence of mirror artifact excludes pathology, such as fluid behind the diaphragm (**Fig. 31**).

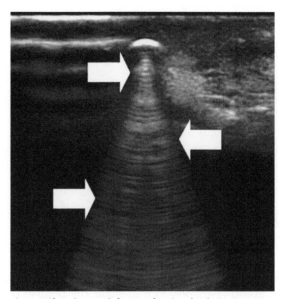

Fig. 28. Reverberation artifact (*arrows*) from a foreign body in tissue.

DOPPLER

Doppler imaging is an integral part of an ultrasound examination. Doppler imaging is used to examine the flow of blood, in particular the direction, velocity, and pattern of blood flow through the organ of interest. When discussing Doppler, it is important to

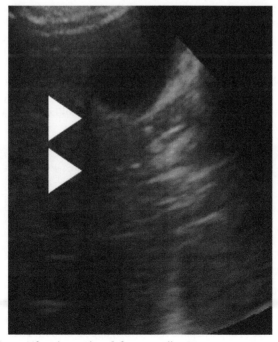

Fig. 29. Shadowing artifact (*arrowhead*) from a gallstone.

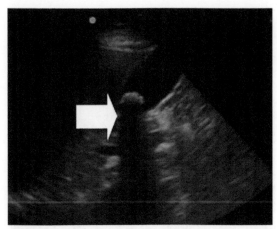

Fig. 30. Edge artifact (*arrow*) from a gall bladder wall.

remember the difference between velocity and speed. Velocity is magnitude plus direction, whereas speed refers only to magnitude The Doppler principle is based on the perceived pitch of sound. A sound source moving toward the listener appears to have a higher pitch, whereas, a sound source moving away from the listener appears to have a lower pitch. This difference, or shift, in frequency is the Doppler frequency.[2]

In diagnostic ultrasound, Doppler shifts are created when transmitted sound waves strike moving red blood cells (**Figs. 32** and **33**). When red blood cells move toward the transducer, the Doppler frequency is higher than the transmitted frequency (positive shift). When red blood cells move away from the transducer, the Doppler frequency is lower than the transmitted frequency (negative shift). Doppler shifts depend on the velocity of the blood cells. A faster velocity has a greater shift in the Doppler frequency. The equation in **Fig. 32** shows the dependent variables for the Doppler frequency.

The equation shows that the velocity is inversely related to the transducer frequency and points out a few important distinctions. As discussed previously, a higher transducer frequency is desirable because it is associated with a higher resolution. With

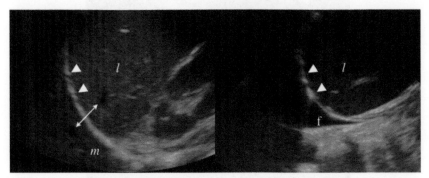

Fig. 31. Mirror artifact in the right upper quadrant. (*Left*) Mirror artifact (m) in a normal patient. Notice liver tissue (l) and a hepatic vein (*arrow*) appear on both sides of the diaphragm (*arrowheads*). (*Right*) Pleural fluid (f) obliterates the artifact.

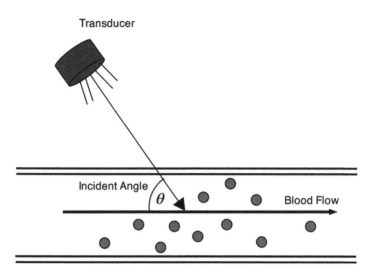

Transducer

Incident Angle

θ

Blood Flow

$$\text{Doppler Shift} = \frac{2 \, x \, v \, x \, F \, x \cos \theta}{\text{Propagation Speed}}$$

Fig. 32. Schematic of the Doppler frequency and the Doppler equation. The transducer sends sound waves at a nonperpendicular angle to the flow of blood in a blood vessel.

Doppler imaging, a lower frequency is better because it allows high flow velocity to be measured. Faster velocities can be measured with lower frequency. Another fact from the diagram and equation (see **Fig. 32**) is that the incident angle is important. Because the cosine of a perpendicular angle is 0, no Doppler shift can be recorded at a perpendicular incidence to flow. Conversely, the greatest shift can be recorded parallel to flow.

There are different types of Doppler that are used in standard diagnostic imaging. The two most common are continuous wave Doppler and pulsed Doppler. As the

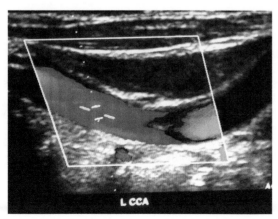

Fig. 33. Doppler image. Note the cursor (aka gate) at the level of the vessel. Angled incidence is measured. No measurements can be made at a perpendicular angle. (*Courtesy of* Christine Birch, RDCS, Cardiac Sonographer, Phoenix, AZ.)

name suggests, continuous wave Doppler requires 1 crystal to transmit continuously and 1 to receive continuously. Continuous wave Doppler can accurately record high velocities. It cannot, however, determine exact locations of a moving red blood cell.

In pulsed wave Doppler, only 1 crystal is required because it can both transmit and pause to receive signals in-between pulses. In this case, a sonographer positions a sample volume (cursor or gate) on an image. The amount of time to transmit and reflect a pulse is calculated corresponding to the depth of the sample volume. Pulsed wave Doppler, however, is inaccurate in the measurement of high-velocity signals (aka aliasing).

BIOEFFECTS

When discussing the physics of diagnostic ultrasound, it is important to mention bioeffects. As discussed previously, intensities of sound are important in determining bioeffects of ultrasound on human tissue. Because it is known that bone absorbs ultrasound waves, there are slight temperature elevations expected at the interface between tissue and bone. The American Institute of Ultrasound in Medicine compiles safety information on the use of ultrasound based on the current available literature. They state, "There are no confirmed biological effects on patients or instrument operators caused by exposures from present diagnostic ultrasound instruments…current data indicate that the benefits to patients of the prudent use of diagnostic ultrasound outweigh the risks, if any, that may be present."[3]

That said, the potential benefits and risks of each examination should be considered. The principle, as low as reasonably achievable, should be observed when performing diagnostic medical ultrasound. Pulsed Doppler has the highest output intensities, and gray scale (B-mode) imaging has the lowest output intensities. Finally, examination duration has the greatest effect on patient exposure.[3]

SUMMARY

In conclusion, point-of-care or bedside ultrasound is an important addition to the way patients are examined, diagnosed, and managed. Its utility at the bedside is just now being recognized. Understanding the physics of sound waves and how the system generate images is important in acquiring the best possible images to aid in diagnosis and management.

REFERENCES

1. Zagzebski JA. Essentials of ultrasound physics. Mosby; 1996.
2. Edelman SK. Understanding ultrasound physics. ESP; 2005.
3. American Institute of ultrasound in Medicine medical ultrasound safety. American Institute of Ultrasound in Medicine; 2009.
4. Gibbs V, Cole D, Sassano A. Ultrasound physics and technology: how, why and when. Elsevier Health Sciences; 2009.
5. Armstrong WF, Ryan T, Feigenbaum H. Feigenbaum's echocardiography. Wolters Kluwer Health/Lippincott Williams & Wilkins; 2010.

An Introduction to Ultrasound Equipment and Knobology

J. Luis Enriquez, MD[a],*, Teresa S. Wu, MD[b]

KEYWORDS

- Ultrasound • Equipment • Knobology • Probes • Transducers • Doppler • B-mode
- M-mode

KEY POINTS

- The use of ultrasonography in medical practice has evolved dramatically over the last few decades and will continue to improve as technological advances are incorporated into daily medical practice.
- Although ultrasound machine size and equipment have evolved, the basic principles and fundamental functions have remained essentially the same.
- Becoming familiar with the machine and the controls used for image generation optimizes the scans being performed and enhances the use of ultrasound in patient care.

INTRODUCTION

The use of ultrasonography in medical practice has evolved dramatically over the last few decades and will continue to improve as technological advances are incorporated into daily medical practice. Although ultrasound (US) machine size and equipment have changed over time, the basic principles and fundamental functions have remained essentially the same. This article reviews the general US apparatus design, the most common probe types available, and the system controls used to manipulate the images obtained. A detailed discussion of the physics involved in medical ultrasonography is presented elsewhere in this issue of *Critical Care Clinics*.

US MACHINES

The fundamental principle of ultrasonography can be traced to approximately 200 years ago when Lazzaro Spallanzani, an Italian biologist, theorized that bats used echolocation to hunt in the dark.[1] During the late 1800s, the concept of sound

The authors have no conflicts of interest or disclosures.
[a] Department of Emergency Medicine, Maricopa Medical Center, 2601 East Roosevelt Street, Phoenix, AZ 85008, USA; [b] EM Residency Program, Emergency Medicine, Maricopa Medical Center, University of Arizona, College of Medicine-Phoenix, 2601 East Roosevelt Street, Phoenix, AZ 85008, USA
* Corresponding author.
E-mail address: jlenriquez55@yahoo.com

was expressed mathematically by the English physicist Lord Raleigh.[2] In 1880, the piezoelectric effect of crystals was first described by Pierre and Jacques Curie.[3] These principles in physics were initially incorporated into industrial applications (eg, identifying structural metal flaws) and eventually were applied in medical practice.[1] The first known published medical US application was in 1942 by the Viennese brothers, Karl and Friederich Dussik.[1] It was not until 1963 that the first real-time commercial US machine became available by Vidoson Siemens, Corp.

Almost 50 years after the first bulky US machine made its debut, compact and portable US machines started making their way into standard bedside use. Many of the popular US machines being used in patient care areas are no larger than small laptop computers. As technology continues to evolve at a dramatic pace, there are US machines being developed that are comparable with the size of an average cellular phone (**Figs. 1** and **2**).[4–6] Furthermore, there are applications for actual smart phones that connect to a scanning probe enabling the operator to perform ultrasonography without an actual US machine (**Fig. 3**).

The discussion here is limited to the compact, laptop size US machines used most frequently for point-of-care (POC) scans in the acute care setting. There are a variety of US machine brands (**Figs. 4–6**) available for POC US at the bedside. All of the machines include a user interface with a keyboard and, depending on the brand, a variety of knobs, buttons, track ball, or touch screen for manipulation and storage of the images. Deciding which US machine to purchase for POC scans depends not only on the price of the machine, but also its durability, the life span of the battery, need for AC energy, boot-up time, portability, and previous experience with a particular US machine brand.

Most of the US machines for POC use are attached to a cart that not only provides a base for the machine itself, but also facilitates portability to different areas of the department and hospital. These carts also have the space to store different probes, cables for AC connection, sterile probe covers, bottles of gel, and other supplies that can be used as needed during the scans (**Fig. 7**).

A secondary viewing screen can be attached to the cart, above the main US screen. This secondary screen can be used for patient viewing or for bedside teaching (**Fig. 8**).

US PROBES

Although there are many US transducers designed for specific uses in medical practice, most of POC ultrasonography can be accomplished using one of four basic types of probes: (1) curvilinear, (2) linear, (3) sector/phased, and (4) intracavity (**Figs. 9–12**).

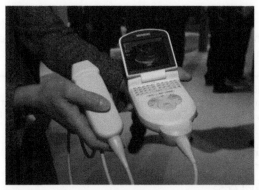

Fig. 1. Portable handheld ultrasound machine Acuson P-10. (*Courtesy of* Siemens Healthcare Copyright 2013; with permission.)

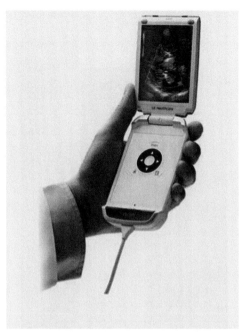

Fig. 2. Vscan handheld ultrasound. (*Courtesy of* General Electric Healthcare; with permission.)

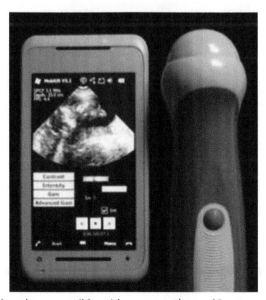

Fig. 3. Ultrasound probe compatible with a smart phone. (*Courtesy of* Mobil US; with permission.)

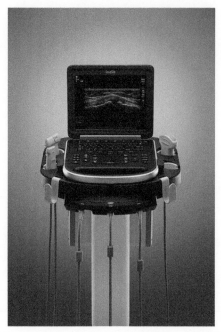

Fig. 4. SonoSite bedside ultrasound machine. (*Courtesy of* FUJIFILM Sonosite Inc; with permission.)

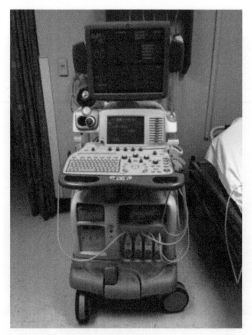

Fig. 5. General Electric bedside ultrasound machine.

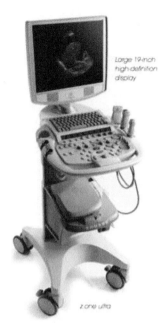

Fig. 6. Zonare bedside ultrasound machine. (*Courtesy of* Zonare Medical Systems Inc; with permission.)

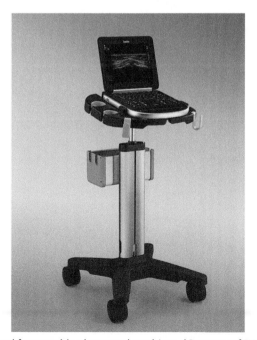

Fig. 7. Universal stand for portable ultrasound machines. (*Courtesy of* FUJIFILM Sonosite Inc; with permission.)

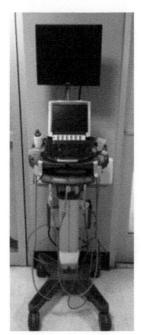

Fig. 8. Ultrasound machine with teaching or secondary viewing screen mounted on the portable stand.

The basic US transducer is composed of the head, the wire, and the connector. In most machines, the transducer is interchangeable by detaching it completely from the US machine base. Many POC US machines can be fitted with a transducer connector that allows practitioners to select the appropriate probe for a study by simply pressing

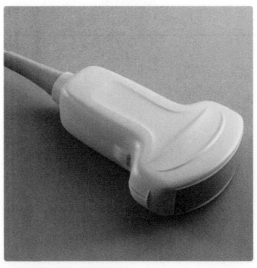

Fig. 9. Low-frequency curvilinear transducer.

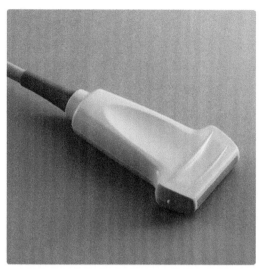

Fig. 10. High-frequency linear array transducer.

a button or touching the probe icon on a screen. These transducer connectors enable rapid interchangeability between probes without having to detach them individually from the US machine (**Fig. 13**).

Technology is advancing rapidly and, by the end of 2012, Siemens Corporation unveiled the first wireless US probe. Having a cordless US probe is beneficial in preventing cord entanglement and potentially allowing for more mobility and range of movement during a bedside scan. The disadvantages include risk of misplacing or losing the cordless probe, and interface malfunctions between the signal from the probe and the US machine.

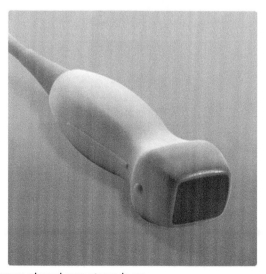

Fig. 11. Low-frequency phased array transducer.

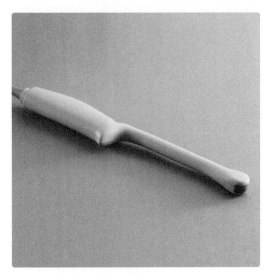

Fig. 12. Higher-frequency intracavitary transducer.

When discussing the general US equipment that is used for POC scans, it is important to know the standard names given to the various parts of the machine and probes.[7,8] The tip of the probe head is referred to as the footprint. The footprint is the part of the probe that is in direct contact with the patient through an acoustic

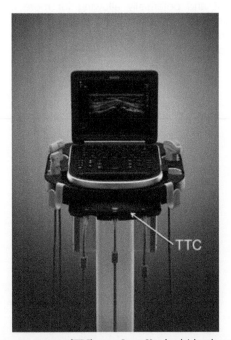

Fig. 13. Triple transducer connector (TTC) on a SonoSite bedside ultrasound machine. (*Courtesy of* FUJIFILM Sonosite Inc; with permission.)

window (eg, US gel). Larger footprints provide a more expansive scanning area. Smaller footprints are preferred for examinations that require maneuvering of the probe in smaller anatomic regions (eg, intercostal spaces in pediatric patients, fontanels, cardiac examinations, and so forth). The type of scan being performed and individual patient characteristics determine which footprint is best suited for image acquisition.

Piezoelectric crystals are located at the footprint of the probe and, except for the sector probe, they are arranged according to the shape of the probe tip. The footprint is a transmitter and receiver of the US beam during scanning. Most modern probes use synthetic plumbium zirconium titanate, compared with quartz crystals that were used in earlier units. These plumbium zirconium titanate crystals are integral in the image quality obtained during the scan, and can be damaged or misaligned when probes are dropped, crushed, or thrown against other objects.

Every US probe should have a probe marker along one side of the head of the probe. This marker can be a colored light, dot, or a linear ridge that can be easily palpated while handling the probe (**Fig. 14**). This marker becomes important for orientation of the patient's anatomy in relationship to the maker displayed on the US machine screen (**Fig. 15**). In standard practice, this orientation marker should be pointed toward either the patient's right side or the patient's head during the scan. The exceptions to this rule occur during scans of a patient's internal jugular vein during a central venous access cannulation, and during some of the cardiac views (discussed elsewhere in this issue).

The fundamental principle of tissue penetration of the ultrasonic beam, expressed in megahertz, determines the type of transducer that should be used. Higher-frequency probes provide less penetration of the US waves through the tissue planes, but generate higher-resolution images. High-frequency probes should be used to visualize superficial structures, such as tendons, muscle, pulmonary pleura, vasculature, and so forth. Conversely, probes with a lower spectrum of frequency should be used to visualize deeper structures. The ability to visualize deeper structures comes at the expense of resolution. Lower-frequency probes are useful in evaluating the abdominal aorta, the gallbladder, the inferior vena cava (IVC), pelvic organs, and so forth.

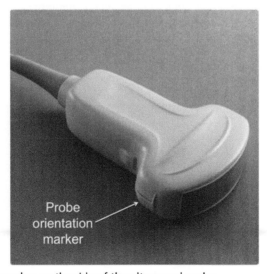

Fig. 14. Indicator marker on the side of the ultrasound probe.

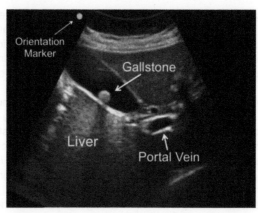

Fig. 15. Orientation marker on the left side of the ultrasound image.

The curvilinear or convex array probe (**Fig. 16**) has a frequency range of 2 to 5 MHz. It provides a wide, fan-shaped scanning area on the US screen. This type of transducer is mostly used for evaluating deep structures in the abdomen and pelvis. Common clinical scenarios for this type of probe are patients with abdominal pain to evaluate for abdominal aortic aneurysm or gallbladder pathology, abdominal pain in pregnancy,[9] or the focused assessment with sonography in trauma (FAST examination).[10]

The intracavitary probe also has a curvilinear crystal array with a wide view. However, the frequency is much higher (8–13 MHz) than other curved probes. Because of the higher frequency, the resolution of the images is better. Examples of applications with this probe are oral pathology (eg, peritonsillar abscess)[11] and transvaginal pelvic evaluations (eg, ovarian torsion, pregnancy, and so forth) (**Fig. 17**).

The linear transducer has a rectangular footprint shape with a frequency range of 6 to 15 MHz (**Fig. 18**). This probe provides detailed anatomic resolution and is ideal for evaluating superficial structures. A wide variety of pathology can be seen at the bedside with this type of probe, such as deep venous thrombosis,[12] musculoskeletal trauma,[13] subcutaneous foreign bodies and abscesses,[14] testicular torsion,[15] pneumothorax,[16] and ocular pathology.[17,18] The linear array probe can also be used to guide such procedures as venous access (central and peripheral);[19] arthrocentesis; needle aspirations; and lumbar punctures.[20]

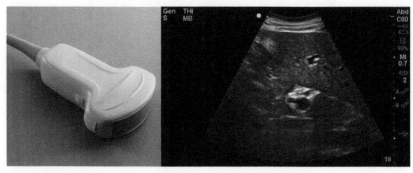

Fig. 16. Curvilinear probe and corresponding ultrasound image.

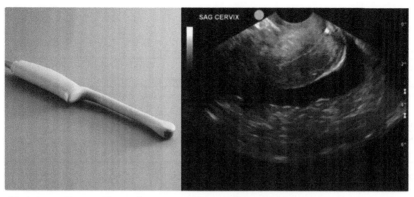

Fig. 17. Intracavitary probe and corresponding ultrasound image.

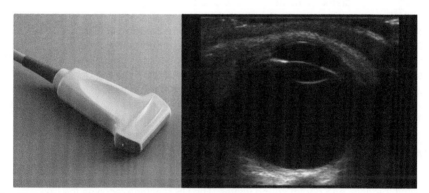

Fig. 18. Linear array transducer and corresponding ultrasound image.

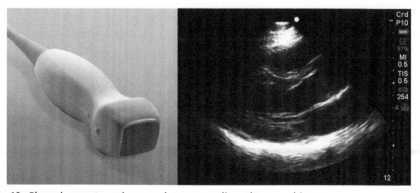

Fig. 19. Phased array transducer and corresponding ultrasound image.

Table 1 Transducer type and clinical use		
Probe Type	**Frequency (MHz)**	**Applications**
Curvilinear	2–5	FAST, renal, aorta, IVC, pelvic, bladder, bowel, appendicitis
Linear	6–15	Ocular, trachea, thyroid, thoracic, vascular access, DVT, MSK, soft tissue, appendicitis
Intracavitary	8–13	Peritonsillar abscess, pelvic
Phased array/sector	1–5	Cardiac, abdominal, renal, pediatric abdomen, bladder, bowel, IVC

Abbreviations: DVT, deep venous thrombosis; FAST, focused assessment with sonography in trauma; IVC, inferior vena cava; MSK, musculoskeletal.

The phased or sector array transducer has a frequency range of 1 to 5 MHz. The crystal arrangement in the footprint is bundled in the center and fans out creating a pielike image on the US machine screen (**Fig. 19**). Because of the smaller footprint, this probe is commonly used for echocardiography and is particularly useful in the evaluation of pediatric patients.[21,22] The phased array probe can also be used for the FAST examination in patients with tight intercostal spaces. The most commonly used US probes and beside US applications are summarized in **Table 1**.

Some US machines allow the user to change the broadband frequency used during the scan. For example, when using a multifrequency transducer, it is useful to be able to scan at the lower or higher ends of the probe frequency. On the US machine, there may be image optimization controls that allow the user to increase penetration (scan at a lower frequency); increase resolution (scan at a higher frequency); or scan in general settings (between the highest and lowest frequency available).

IMAGE PRODUCTION AND SYSTEM CONTROLS

To produce US images for evaluation, the machine and probes work in concert to transmit, receive, and depict sound waves. The US machine receives the beam signal as amplitude, frequency, and the changes of the frequency over time. The two-dimensional gray scale of the image is generated from the amplitude of the echoes. The change of the frequency and wavelength of the US echoes from a target in motion is known as the Doppler effect. Further information about the physics of bedside US can be found in elsewhere in this issue.

Before beginning a scan, it is important to set up the US machine for the type of scan being performed. Most modern-day US machines have standard presets for common applications (eg, abdomen, obstetrics, vascular, musculoskeletal). These presets can be selected by a menu available on the US machine, and are often programmable based on the user's preferences.

During the scan, real-time images of the tissue anatomy and motion can be obtained in B-mode scanning, M-mode scanning, and with Doppler. B-mode, otherwise known as "brightness" mode, displays a two-dimensional, gray scale image on the screen. The gray scale of the image can be manipulated by adjusting the gain (**Figs. 20–22**). By increasing the gain, the US machine allows processing of more incoming echoes, thereby creating a brighter image. A darker image is obtained when the gain is decreased (see **Fig. 22**). Gain can be adjusted in the nearfield, farfield, or overall field of the screen display. Increasing the gain leads to a brighter image on the screen, but it also increases image noise and artifact, with loss of contrast and finer details.

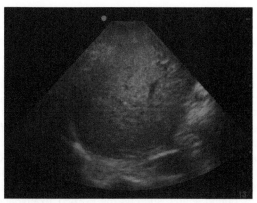

Fig. 20. Evaluation of the liver with increased gain.

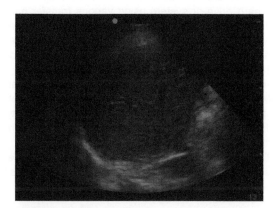

Fig. 21. Evaluation of the liver with normal gain.

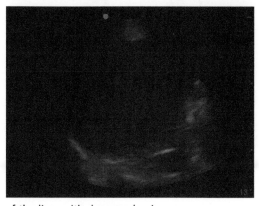

Fig. 22. Evaluation of the liver with decreased gain.

As the US beam travels deeper into a medium, the returning echoes are attenuated, resulting in less resolution. A feature known as time gain compensation allows the sonographer to adjust the image brightness at specific depths. The top row of buttons controls nearfield gain, whereas the bottom row of buttons controls farfield gain (**Fig. 23**). Advanced US machines may also have an "auto gain" button, which resets the machine back to standard gain presets for the type of scan being performed.

Most US machines allow the user to freeze and save still images and to capture video clips (**Fig. 24**). Having the ability to freeze an image on the US screen becomes important when measurements are being obtained, or fine details of a scan are being examined. These still images can be saved or printed for further review and archiving.

The ability to obtain video clips is another useful function of modern day US machines. Video clips are most often used in documenting cardiac wall motion; in monitoring needle trajectory during US-guided procedures; and evaluating dynamic movement of organs during scans, such as the E-FAST examination. The length of the video clips can be manually adjusted using standard control buttons and options on the machine. The format of the video clips differs depending on the manufacturer presets (eg, .mov, .mp4).

The still images or video clips can be stored on the US machine hard drive or transferred to a remote hard drive or system using various transfer methods. Most machines allow for the transfer of data by USB ports, FireWire, expansion cards, Ethernet ports, or wireless portals. Newer US machines are equipped to transmit images for review and storage on systems with digital imaging and communication in medicine (DICOM) capabilities.

In addition to B-mode capabilities, most machines also allow scanning in M-mode ("motion" mode). M-mode obtains an image in the B-mode and displays it graphically as changes over a period of time. Useful applications for this modality include assessment of the IVC for intravascular volume, estimating wall movement and cardiac contractility, and the evaluation of a pneumothorax (**Fig. 25**).

The use of the Doppler principle in POC ultrasonography includes color Doppler, pulse wave Doppler, and color power Doppler. Color Doppler detects the overall blood

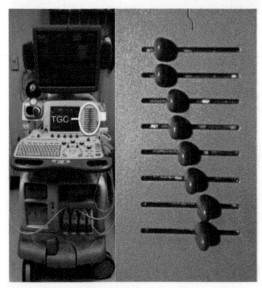

Fig. 23. Time gain compensation (TGC) control.

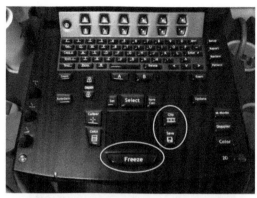

Fig. 24. Freeze, save, and video clip buttons on an ultrasound machine.

flow and its direction of flow under a region of interrogation (eg, identification of vessels close to an abscess before incision, or turbulent flow in an abdominal aortic aneurysm) (**Fig. 26**). The energy of the returning echoes is displayed as an assigned color on the US screen. By convention, echoes demonstrating flow toward the transducer are seen in shades of red. Those representing flow away from the transducer are seen as shades of blue. The color display is usually superimposed on the B-mode image, thus allowing simultaneous visualization of anatomy and flow dynamics.

In pulse wave Doppler, the direction and velocity of the blood flow can be displayed graphically and audibly (**Fig. 27**). If blood is moving away from the transducer, a lower frequency (negative shift) is detected. If blood is moving toward the transducer, a higher frequency (positive shift) is detected. This Doppler modality also provides information about laminar versus turbulent flow (eg, flow within an abdominal aortic aneurysm).

Color power Doppler identifies the amplitude or power of the Doppler signals rather than the frequency shifts. It is more sensitive than pulse wave Doppler to detect blood flow in organs with typically low-flow states, such as the ovaries or testicles. Color power Doppler is particularly useful in the evaluation of ovarian or testicular torsion (**Fig. 28**).

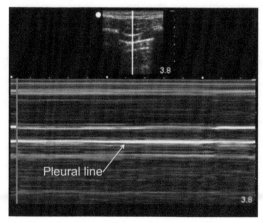

Fig. 25. M-mode evaluation of a pneumothorax. (*Courtesy of* Teresa Wu, MD, Associate Professor, Emergency Medicine, University of Arizona, College of Medicine-Phoenix, Phoenix, AZ.)

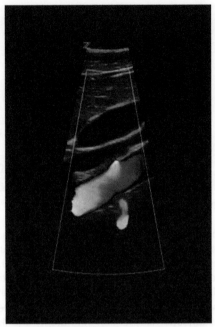

Fig. 26. Color Doppler flow through the aorta farfield to the IVC and gallbladder. (*Courtesy of* Zonare Medical Systems Inc; with permission.)

OBTAINING CALCULATIONS ON BEDSIDE US

During bedside scans, it is often useful to obtain specific measurements of the structure being evaluated. For example, measurements of the IVC diameter are being used to guide resuscitation attempts (**Fig. 29**). Most machines have a caliper button that allows the user to measure the absolute distance between two points. The select key is typically used to toggle between the two calipers. Once both calipers have been aligned along the border of the object being measured, the distance between the calipers is displayed on the US screen (**Fig. 30**).

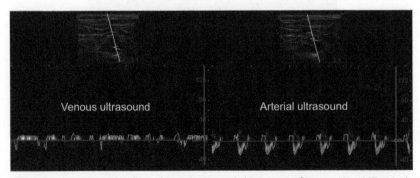

Fig. 27. Pulse wave Doppler flow through a vessel. (*Courtesy of* Teresa Wu, MD, Maricopa Medical Center, University of Arizona, College of Medicine-Phoenix, Phoenix, AZ.)

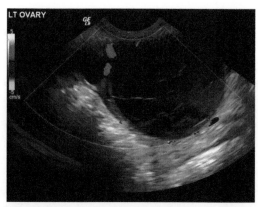

Fig. 28. Evaluation of ovarian torsion using color Doppler. (*Courtesy of* Mary Connell, MD, Department of Radiology, Maricopa Medical Center, Phoenix, AZ.)

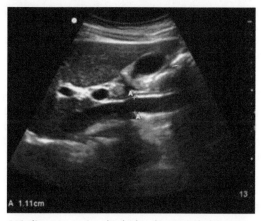

Fig. 29. Measuring IVC diameter using bedside ultrasound. (*Courtesy of* Teresa Wu, MD, Maricopa Medical Center, University of Arizona, College of Medicine-Phoenix, Phoenix, AZ.)

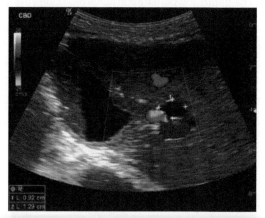

Fig. 30. Using the calipers to calculate the diameter of an enlarged common bile duct. Note that the dimensions of the common bile duct are shown in the bottom left side of the image (0.92 × 1.29 cm). (*Courtesy of* Teresa Wu, MD, Maricopa Medical Center, University of Arizona, College of Medicine-Phoenix, Phoenix, AZ.)

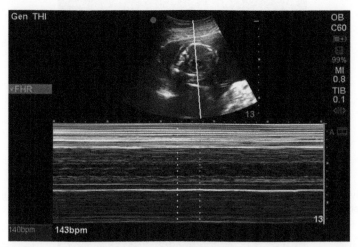

Fig. 31. Obtaining fetal heart rate using the calculations option during a bedside obstetric ultrasound. (*Courtesy of* Teresa Wu, MD, Maricopa Medical Center, University of Arizona, College of Medicine-Phoenix, Phoenix, AZ.)

Many US machines have preset calculations available for the particular imaging mode or examination type being used. For example, if an obstetric US is being performed, common preset calculations include fetal heart rate, crown rump length, biparietal diameter, and head circumference. Selecting the desired calculation from the available menu provides automatic calculations of the region being measured (**Fig. 31**).

ADJUSTING THE DEPTH OF THE SCAN

The penetration of the US beam on a particular transducer can be altered by manipulating the frequency of the probe and adjusting the depth or penetration button/knob on the US machine. The depth and penetration achieved during the scan are displayed

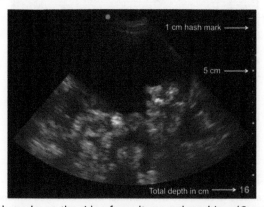

Fig. 32. Depth hash marks on the side of an ultrasound machine. (*Courtesy of* Teresa Wu, MD, Maricopa Medical Center, University of Arizona, College of Medicine-Phoenix, Phoenix, AZ.)

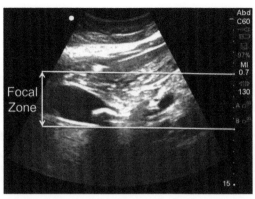

Fig. 33. Adjust the depth of the scan so that the target structure is visualized within the "focal zone" (middle and narrowest portion of the ultrasound beam). (*Courtesy of* Teresa Wu, MD, Maricopa Medical Center, University of Arizona, College of Medicine-Phoenix, Phoenix, AZ.)

as a scale on the left or right side of the US screen. By convention, these hash marks are designated at 0.1-, 0.5-, and 1-cm increments (**Fig. 32**). During the initial part of a scan, it is often useful to start with an increased depth for orientation purposes and to evaluate surrounding structures. Once the target structure has been localized, scanning depth should be decreased to minimize the display of irrelevant deeper structures. Scanning at increased depths reduces the frame rate and compromises image quality.

In between the nearfield and farfield of the US beam is what is known as the "focal zone." This is the narrowest part of the beam and provides the greatest lateral resolution during the scan. It is important to manually adjust the depth of the scan so that the target structure is visualized within the focal zone of the US beam (**Fig. 33**).

Many advanced US systems also provide the option to zoom in on or magnify an area of particular interest. By zooming in on an object, the US field and processing is restricted to that particular target area and assigned to the image matrix. Pressing the zoom button on the US machine brings up a box on the screen. Using the track

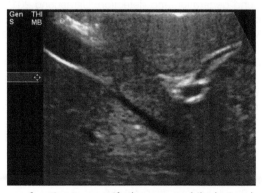

Fig. 34. Using the zoom function to magnify the common bile duct and portal vein for analysis. (*Courtesy of* Teresa Wu, MD, Maricopa Medical Center, University of Arizona, College of Medicine-Phoenix, Phoenix, AZ.)

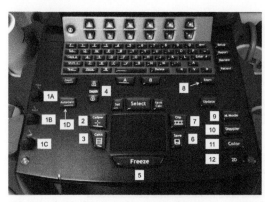

1A: Nearfield gain
1B: Farfield gain
1C: Overall gain
1D: Auto gain
2: Calipers
3: Calculations
4: Depth
5: Freeze
6: Save (for still images)
7: Clip (to save video clips)
8: Exam (to select exam types)
9: M Mode
10: Pulse Wave Doppler
11: Color Doppler
12: 2D (B Mode)

Fig. 35. Standard ultrasound controls, buttons, and knobs.

pad, this magnification box can be maneuvered over the area of interest. Pressing the zoom button again enlarges the area that has been selected (**Fig. 34**).

SUMMARY

Understanding basic US instrumentation and knobology is an important step in learning how to perform bedside US examinations. Although US machines may differ in some of their capabilities, the standard instrumentation and functionality remain essentially the same (**Fig. 35**). Becoming familiar with the machine and the controls used for image generation optimizes the scans being performed and enhances the use of US in patient care.

REFERENCES

1. Hoffman B, Nixon MS. Ultrasound guide for emergency physicians. An introduction. physics and technical facts for the beginner. 2008. Available at: http://sonoguide.com/physics.htlm. Accessed January 3, 2013.
2. Rayleigh Lord. The theory of sound. Cambridge: University Press; 2011.
3. Manbachi A, Cobbold RSC. Development and application of pizoelectric materials for ultrasound generation and detection. Ultrasound 2011;19(4):187–96.
4. Kendall JL, Hoffenberg SR, Smith S. History of emergency and critical care ultrasound: The evolution of a new imaging paradigm. Critical Care Med 2007;35: S126–30.
5. Lapostolle F, Petrovic T, Lenoir G, et al. Usefulness of hand-held ultrasound devices in out-of-hospital diagnosis performed by emergency physicians. Am J Emerg Med 2006;24(2):237–42.
6. Blaivas M, Brannam L, Theodoro D. Ultrasound image quality comparison between an inexpensive hand-held emergency department (ED) ultrasound machine and a large mobile ED ultrasound system. Acad Emerg Med 2004;11(7):778–81.
7. Brull R, McFarlane AJ, Tse CC. Practical knobology for ultrasound-guided regional anesthesia. Reg Anesth Pain Med 2010;35:S68–73.
8. Ihnatsenka B, Boezaart AP. Ultrasound: Basic understanding and learning the language. Int J Shoulder Surg 2010;4(3):55–62.
9. Emergency ulrasound imaging criteria compendium. American College of Emergency Physicians. Ann Emerg Med 2009;53:550–70.

10. American Institute of Ultrasound in Medicine. AIUM practice guidelines for the performance of the focussed assessment with sonography for trauma (FAST) examination. J Ultraound Med 2008;27(2):313–8.
11. Lyon M, Blaivas M. Intraoral ultrasound in the diagnosis and treatment of suspected peritonsillar abscess in the emergency department. Acad Emerg Med 2005;12(1):85–8.
12. Kline JA, O'Malley PM, Tayal VS, et al. Emergency clinician-performed compressed ultrasonography for deep venous thrombosis of the lower extremity. Ann Emerg Med 2008;52:437–45.
13. Marshburn TH, Legone E, Sargysan A, et al. Goal-directed ultrasound in the detection of long bone fractures. J Trauma 2004;57(2):329–32.
14. Chau CL, Griffith JF. Musculoskeletal infections: ultrasound appearance. Clin Radiol 2005;60(2):149–59.
15. Blaivas M, Sierzenski P, Lambert M. Emergency evaluation of patients presenting with acute scrotum using bedside ultrasonography. Acad Emerg Med 2001;8: 90–3.
16. Lichenstein DA, Mexiere G, Lascolis N, et al. Ultrasound diagnosis of occult pneumothorax. Critical Care Med 2005;33:1231–8.
17. Kimberly HH, Shah S, Marill K, et al. Correlation of optic nerve sheath diameter with direct measurement of intracranial pressure. Acad Emerg Med 2008;15: 201–4.
18. Le A, Hoehn ME, Spentzas T, et al. Bedside sonographic measurements of ocular nerve sheath diameter as a predictor of increased intracranial pressure in children. Ann Emerg Med 2009;53:785–91.
19. Troianos AC, Hartman SG, Glas EK, et al. Guidelines for performing ultrasound guided vascular cannulation. J Am Soc Echocardiogr 2011;24:1291–318.
20. Ferre RM, Sweeney TW. Emergency physicians can easily obtain ultrasound images of anatomical landmarks relevant to lumbar puncture. Am J Emerg Med 2007;25(3):291–6.
21. Elavunkal J, Bright L, Stone MB. Emergency ultrasound identification of loculated pericardial effusion: The importance of multiple cardiac views. Acad Emerg Med 2010;39(5):637–43.
22. Pershad J, Meyer S, Plouman C, et al. Bedside limited echocardiography by the emergency physician is accurate during evaluation of the critically ill patient. Pediatrics 2004;114(6):e667–71.

Cardiac Echocardiography

Phillips Perera, MD, RDMS*, Viveta Lobo, MD, Sarah R. Williams, MD,
Laleh Gharahbaghian, MD

KEYWORDS

- Cardiac echocardiography • Focused echocardiography
- Bedside echocardiography • Cardiac ultrasound • Pericardial effusion
- Cardiac tamponade • Cardiac contractility • Pulmonary embolism

KEY POINTS

- Focused cardiac echocardiography has become a critical diagnostic tool for both the emergency physician and critical care physician caring for patients with chest pain, shortness of breath, in a shock state or following trauma to the chest.
- Cardiac echocardiography allows for the immediate diagnosis of pericardial effusions and cardiac tamponade, the evaluation of cardiac contractility and volume status, and the detection of right ventricular strain that may be seen with a significant pulmonary embolus.
- Advanced echocardiography applications that utilize Doppler technology may be used for more advanced ultrasonographic examinations (cardiac valvular, hemodynamic evaluations).
- The emergent cardiac procedures, pericardiocentesis and placement of a transvenous pacemaker wire, can be performed more accurately and safely with ultrasound guidance.
- This article covers how to perform cardiac echocardiography using the standard windows, how to interpret a focused goal-directed examination, and how to apply this information clinically at the bedside.

INTRODUCTION

Cardiac echocardiography has evolved to become one of the most important clinical skills for both the emergency physician (EP) and the critical care physician (CCP). Current ultrasound technology contained in smaller and more portable units has dramatically improved in the recent past to allow for performance of focused echocardiography in the relative safety of monitored clinical areas.[1] Essential treatment of the

Funding Sources: All authors disclose no funding sources.
Conflicts of Interest: Phillips Perera is an educational consultant for Sonosite Ultrasound. All other authors disclose no conflicts of interest.
Division of Emergency Medicine, Department of Surgery, Stanford University Medical Center, 300 Pasteur Drive, Alway Building M121, Stanford, CA 94305, USA
* Corresponding author.
E-mail address: pperera1@mac.com

Crit Care Clin 30 (2014) 47–92
http://dx.doi.org/10.1016/j.ccc.2013.08.003
0749-0704/14/$ – see front matter © 2014 Elsevier Inc. All rights reserved.

patient can therefore be rendered concurrently with diagnostic echocardiography. The use of focused ultrasonography has been supported by the major emergency medicine societies, including the American College of Emergency Physicians (ACEP), the Society for Academic Emergency Medicine, and the Council of Residency Directors, all of which currently endorse residency and postresidency training in this modality as well as its clinical use.[2–5] Critical care societies have also endorsed similar guidelines in the use of echocardiography with several consensus documents over the past years.[6–8] In 2010, an important collaborative article was published jointly between the American Society of Echocardiography (ASE) and ACEP, which endorsed focused echocardiography for a defined set of emergent conditions.[9]

GOALS OF FOCUSED BEDSIDE ULTRASONOGRAPHY

The various categories of functional uses, clinical indications, and clinical goals of bedside echocardiography, as defined by ACEP, ASE and Critical Care Medicine guidelines, are summarized in **Tables 1–5**.

PERFORMANCE OF THE ECHOCARDIOGRAPHY EXAMINATION
Selection of Ultrasound Probe

A phased-array probe is typically used for cardiac echocardiography. This probe has the benefit of a small footprint that can easily fit in between the ribs. For the deeper imaging needed for echocardiography, select a frequency at the lower end of the bandwidth used for medical imaging, usually 2.5 to 3 MHz.

Imaging Modalities

Frame rate
As the heart is moving rapidly in reference to other body structures, selection of a high frame rate on the settings of the ultrasound machine will allow for optimal imaging (24 frames per second or higher); this is done by selecting the cardiac preset on the ultrasound machine, which effectively increases the imaging frame rate.

B-mode ultrasonography
Ultrasonography of the heart typically utilizes modalities that can capture both anatomy and physiology[10]; this is done by first using B-mode imaging to visualize the heart as it moves through the cardiac cycle. B-mode imaging projects the heart as a continuum of color in the gray spectrum. Brighter structures are defined as hyperechoic, darker structures as hypoechoic, and the darkest structures as anechoic. Echogenicity results from the fact that the ultrasound probe first acts as a transducer that sends sound waves into the body. The sound waves then penetrate into the body, traveling a distance until they are bounced back to the probe. Different tissue will have varying

---

Table 1
American College of Emergency Physicians functional categories for ultrasonographic examination

ACEP Guidelines for Emergency Ultrasound
Functional categories:
A. Diagnostic
B. Symptom or sign based
C. Therapeutic and monitoring
D. Resuscitative
E. Procedure guidance

Table 2
American College of Emergency Physicians and American Society of Echocardiography consensus guidelines for ultrasonographic examination: clinical indications

ACEP/ASE Consensus Guidelines on Focused Echocardiography
Recognized clinical indications for ultrasonographic examination:
1. Cardiac trauma: Focused assessment with sonography in trauma (FAST) examination
2. Cardiac arrest
3. Hypotension/shock
4. Dyspnea/shortness of breath
5. Chest pain

Table 3
American College of Emergency Physicians and American Society of Echocardiography consensus guidelines for core ultrasonographic examination: clinical goals

ACEP/ASE Consensus Guidelines on Focused Echocardiography
Core echocardiography indications:
1. Assessment for pericardial effusions and pericardial tamponade
2. Assessment of global cardiac systolic function
3. Identification of marked right ventricular and left ventricular enlargement
4. Assessment of intravascular volume
5. Guidance of pericardiocentesis
6. Confirmation of transvenous pacemaker wire placement

Table 4
American College of Emergency Physicians and American Society of Echocardiography consensus guidelines for advanced ultrasonographic examination: examination goals

ACEP/ASE Consensus Guidelines on Focused Echocardiography
The following conditions may be suspected on focused echocardiography (additional imaging should be obtained if possible):
1. Intracardiac masses
2. Cardiac chamber thrombus
3. Regional wall motion abnormalities
4. Endocarditis
5. Aortic dissection

Table 5
Critical care guidelines for advanced ultrasonographic examination: examination goals

Critical Care Medicine Proposed Guidelines for Focused Echocardiography:
The following conditions may be evaluated on focused echocardiography:
1. Evaluation of overall heart chambers and examination for abnormal chamber dimensions
2. Assessment of left ventricular function, both "visual" and "measured"
3. Gross preload estimation of the left ventricle and of the entire heart; evaluation of inferior vena cava size through respiratory variations and collapsibility
4. Evaluation of right ventricular function
5. Assessment for the cardiac findings of pulmonary embolism
6. Evaluation of gross valvular dysfunction
7. Imaging for suspected infective endocarditis
8. Evaluation of intracardiac masses
9. Guidance of pericardiocentesis
10. Guidance of mechanical pacing and assessment of mechanical capture

Data from Neri L, Storti E, Lichtenstein D. Toward an ultrasound curriculum for critical care. Crit Care Med 2007;35(Suppl 5):S290–304.

resistance to the movement of sound, known as impedance. Higher-density (higher-impedance) structures will reflect an increasing amount of the sound back to the probe, resulting in a more hyperechoic appearance (ie, a calcified valve). Fluid-filled structures (lower impedance) will allow for increased propagation of sound through the body, leading to an anechoic appearance (ie, blood in the cardiac chambers, fluid around the heart) (**Fig. 1**).

M-mode ultrasonography
M-mode ultrasonography, or "motion" mode, illustrates an "ice-pick" image of movement across a defined anatomical axis in relation to time. This mode generates a grayscale illustration of movement over time that can be used to easily document motion on a static image. For instance, changes in the size of the inferior vena cava (IVC) with respirations can be well illustrated using M-mode.

Doppler ultrasonography
Doppler ultrasound allows for the evaluation of motion. The detection of motion within the body occurs in direct reference to the relative position of the ultrasound probe, a concept termed the Doppler shift. Structures moving toward the probe will result in a shorter frequency of sound in relation to the transducer's selected frequency, while those moving away will have a longer frequency. The Doppler shift can be interpreted in several imaging modalities described below.

Color-flow Doppler This modality demonstrates directionality of flow both toward and away from the probe, and is often used in advanced echocardiography. The convention is that movement toward the probe is represented as red, with movement away from the probe represented as blue. The scale that displays the color-flow Doppler setting on the left of the ultrasound screen should be set high (around 70 cm/s) to best capture the fast flow of the blood moving through the heart (**Fig. 2**).

The mathematical equation that defines the Doppler shift is directly proportional to the cosine of the imaging angle relating the probe to the object of interest. Practically speaking, this means that imaging with color-flow Doppler (and the other types of Doppler discussed herein) is best performed at as close to a direct plane of 0° from

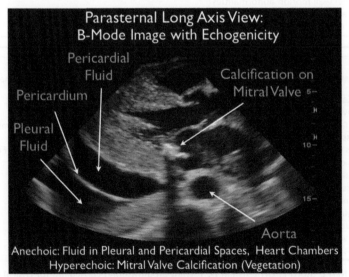

Parasternal Long Axis View: B-Mode Image with Echogenicity

Pericardial Fluid — Pericardium — Pleural Fluid — Calcification on Mitral Valve — Aorta

Anechoic: Fluid in Pleural and Pericardial Spaces, Heart Chambers
Hyperechoic: Mitral Valve Calcification (Vegetation)

Fig. 1. B-mode image, demonstrating spectrum of image echogenicity.

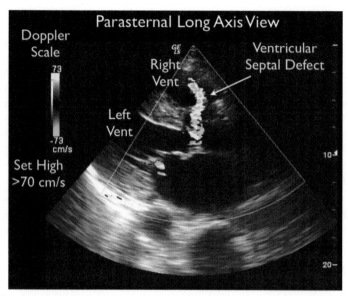

Fig. 2. Color-flow Doppler, with high setting (70 cm/s) for echocardiography.

the probe as possible (cosine of 0 = 1, according the highest Doppler shift). This effectively means that it is best to place the probe as parallel to the direction of blood flow as possible to optimally detect the Doppler signal. The apical view, where blood flow through the heart and the valves is oriented vertically to the path of the sound-waves traveling out from the probe (at close to a 0° configuration), is often the best cardiac window for obtaining the maximal Doppler signal for flow through the cardiac valves.

Pulsed-wave Doppler Pulsed-wave Doppler allows for assessment of the velocity of flow, as indicated in a waveform that identifies the specific speed of blood flow over time. This modality is often used in advanced echocardiography to define the velocity of blood flow through cardiac valves, allowing calculations to be performed for multiple assessments.

Continuous-wave Doppler In this form of Doppler the probe is always on, simultaneously sending sound waves into the body and receiving them as they travel back. This mode differs from pulsed-wave Doppler, during which the probe first transmits sound and then cycles to a receiving mode. Continuous-wave Doppler has definite benefits in echocardiography, as it is not affected by some of the pitfalls of pulsed-wave Doppler technology that may result in a distorted image. One important artifact is aliasing, which will impair the image if the velocity of the sampled column of blood is too high in relation to the pulse frequency of the probe. Continuous-wave Doppler avoids these problems, as it has no upper limit on the detection of the velocity of blood flow. For this reason, it is often used in echocardiography applications that require accurate estimation of the fastest blood flow through the heart.

Probe Versus Ultrasound-Machine Marker Configuration

Historically, there has been practice variation in the orientation of the indicator dot on the screen of the ultrasound machine and the marker on the ultrasound probe. The first widespread applications used in emergency medicine practice, such as the FAST (Focused Assessment with Sonography in Trauma) and obstetrics/gynecology examinations, were oriented based on traditional ultrasonographic protocols for radiology. Emergency focused echocardiography was therefore initially configured similarly to traditional radiology ultrasound practice, with the indicator dot positioned to the left of the ultrasound screen. This configuration differs from traditional cardiology practice whereby the indicator dot was oriented to the right on the screen.

Despite this difference, the standard practice has been to orient the ultrasound probe (at a 180° variance depending on screen orientation) so that the cardiac images obtained following either convention demonstrate the same configuration. In this article, the probe orientation for each cardiac view is described with the ultrasound-screen indicator dot located on the left side.

Standard Echocardiography Windows

There are 3 standard windows for performance of cardiac echocardiography (**Fig. 3**): the parasternal (long-axis and short-axis views), subxiphoid, and apical windows. From each of these windows, variations in the orientation of the probe will allow for additional views to be obtained.

The Parasternal Long-Axis View

The parasternal long-axis view is considered the primary cardiac view by many EPs and CCPs.

Patient position This view can be performed with the patient in a supine position. However, if there is difficulty obtaining a good image, turning the patient into a left lateral decubitus position will often improve the view by moving the heart away from the sternum and closer to the chest wall, thus displacing the lung from the path of the sound waves.

Probe position The probe should be positioned just lateral to the sternum at about the third intercostal space, although one may have to move the probe up or down one intercostal space to achieve the best imaging. The probe indicator should be oriented toward the patient's left elbow (**Fig. 4**).

Because the image depends on aligning the probe along the long axis of the heart, each patient will have a slightly different optimal echocardiographic window. In

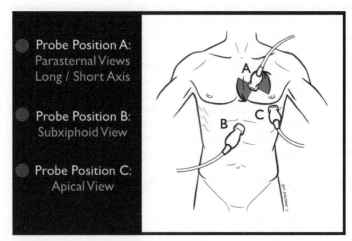

Fig. 3. Cardiac echocardiography, standard windows.

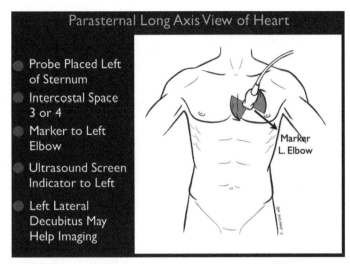

Fig. 4. Parasternal long-axis view: probe position.

patients whose heart may be oriented more vertically, such as those with hyperinflated lungs from asthma and chronic obstructive pulmonary disease (COPD), the probe will need to be aligned correspondingly in a more vertical orientation. The converse occurs in patients with ascites or with other conditions that displace the diaphragms superiorly, for whom the probe orientation will be more horizontal.

Anatomic and sonographic correlation The parasternal long-axis view will visualize the cardiac chambers and the aorta as demonstrated in **Figs. 5** and **6**. This view allows for a detailed evaluation of the left side of the heart, permitting close assessment of chamber sizes and contractility. The right ventricle can also be evaluated from this view. The right atrium is not seen.

The clinician can begin by examination of the left atrium and ventricle. At diastole, a general rule of thumb is that the dimensions of the left atrium should be less than

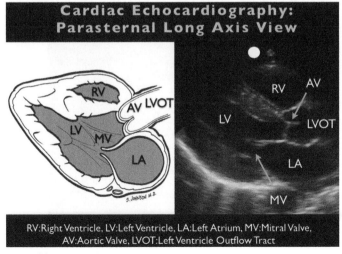

Fig. 5. Parasternal long-axis view: anatomy.

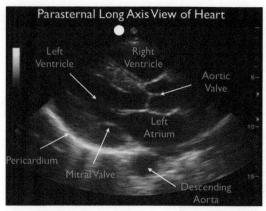

Fig. 6. Descending aorta behind heart.

4.5 cm, and the left ventricle less than 6.0 cm. Hypertrophy of the left ventricular walls can be diagnosed by a wall thickness greater than 10 mm (**Fig. 7**).[11] By contrast, hypertrophy of the right ventricular walls is defined as a wall thickness greater than 5 mm.[11,12]

The aortic valve and aortic root can be visualized as the area known as the left ventricular outflow tract (LVOT). One can examine this area for abnormality of the aortic valve, often indicated by calcifications. A proximal, or Stanford type A aortic dissection may be visualized as a widened aortic root greater than 3.8 cm, measured just distal to the aortic valve (**Fig. 8**).[13] At times an intimal flap may be seen here.[14,15] However, if abnormality of the aorta is highly suspected and is not seen on focused echocardiography, transesophageal echocardiography or computed tomography (CT) imaging would be the usual next diagnostic step.

Imaging tips and tricks Start with the probe position as suggested, with the patient in the left lateral decubitus position. If not able to image the heart from that position, move the probe slightly inferiorly and laterally on the chest wall. The heart may then come into view.

To best image the aortic root, the probe may be moved medially and superiorly from the position where the left ventricle and apex are best visualized. Conversely, moving the probe inferiorly and laterally allows better assessment of the left ventricle. Turning

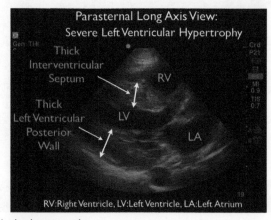

Fig. 7. Left ventricular hypertrophy.

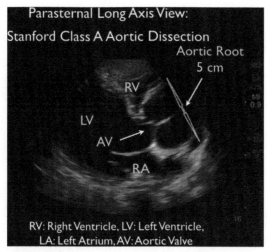

Fig. 8. Proximal aortic dissection.

the probe slightly counterclockwise from the probe position with the indicator oriented to the left elbow may "open up" the left ventricle and allow for a better view of this chamber.

Parasternal Short-Axis View

Probe position This view is obtained by first identifying the heart in the parasternal long-axis view and then swiveling the probe 90° clockwise, so that the indicator dot is aligned toward the patient's right hip (**Fig. 9**).

Anatomic and sonographic correlation The short-axis view is also known as the ring, or doughnut view, and demonstrates the heart in cross section (**Fig. 10**). The classic view is with the probe aligned through the ventricles to capture the mitral valve, which

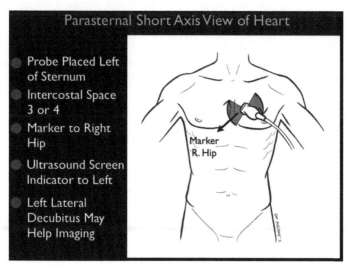

Fig. 9. Parasternal short-axis view: probe position.

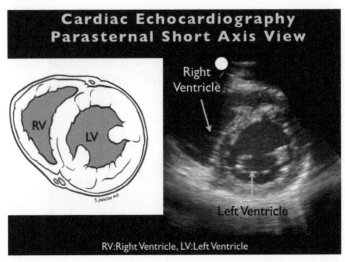

Fig. 10. Parasternal short-axis view: anatomy.

appears as a "fish-mouth" opening and closing in the interior of the ventricle. Visualizing the heart as a cylinder with the ultrasound beam cutting tangentially through different levels, one can look as far inferiorly as the apex of the left ventricle and superiorly to the level of the aortic valve.

To best evaluate the contractions of the left ventricle, the probe is moved inferiorly to image at the level of the papillary muscles. Visual calculations of cardiac contractility can be accurately taken here, confirming the assessment taken from the parasternal long-axis view. In addition, the contractility of specific segments of the left ventricle can be identified, the method through which cardiologists evaluate for segmental wall motion abnormalities.

Imaging tips and tricks The key to finding the optimal window for imaging from the parasternal short-axis view is to first find the best parasternal long-axis window. Once encountered, do not take the probe off the chest. Rotate it 90° clockwise, so the indicator is now oriented to the patient's right hip. The short-axis view should then come into view. The probe can then be moved progressively inferiorly and laterally to view the left ventricle at different levels, all the way down to the apex.

Avoid "overturning" the probe so that the indicator moves increasingly clockwise from the starting orientation toward the right hip. Doing this will convert the parasternal short-axis view into an apical image.

Aortic Valve and Pulmonic Outflow Tract View
Patient position Moving the patient to a left lateral decubitus position is often necessary to best achieve this view.

Probe position This view is a variant of the parasternal short-axis view. If the probe is angled superiorly and medially from the classic view, the aortic valve and pulmonic outflow tract will come into view. The pulmonic outflow tract, consisting of the pulmonary valve and the main pulmonary arteries, can be best seen by aiming the probe slightly lateral from the view of the aortic valve.

Anatomic and sonographic correlation The aortic valve should appear as the "Mercedes-Benz sign" with a normal tricuspid configuration (**Fig. 11**). A calcified bicuspid

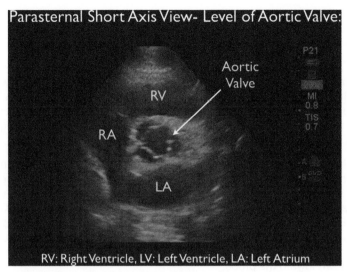

Fig. 11. Parasternal short-axis view: aortic valve.

valve that may be prone to stenosis and abnormality can be identified, often assisted by using the zoom function on the machine.[16] The pulmonic outflow tract can be identified next, just lateral to the aortic valve (**Fig. 12**). Occasionally, saddle pulmonary emboli that sit at the bifurcation of the main pulmonary artery may be seen.[17]

Subxiphoid Window
This view is the classic cardiac window used in the trauma FAST examination.[18]

Patient position This view is usually performed with the patient supine. Having the patient bend the knees may assist in relaxing the abdominal muscles, and improve imaging from this view.

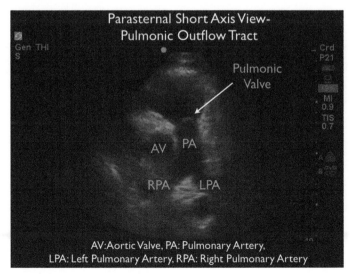

Fig. 12. Parasternal short-axis view: pulmonic outflow.

Probe position The probe is positioned just inferior to the xiphoid tip of the sternum, with the indicator oriented toward the patient's right side (**Fig. 13**). The hand is placed on top of the probe to push it down, so as to aim the ultrasound beam up and under the sternum to image the heart.

Anatomic and sonographic correlation From the subxiphoid view, the liver will act as the acoustic window to the heart, allowing all 4 cardiac chambers to be seen from this position. Because of the superior ability to visualize the right side of the heart from this view, the subxiphoid window is often used when close assessment of right heart chambers is needed (**Fig. 14**).

Imaging tips and tricks The subxiphoid window may offer the best imaging of the heart when the heart is pushed relatively inferiorly, such as in states of hyperinflated lungs (eg, COPD). However, it may be difficult to obtain an adequate view when the gas-filled stomach or intestine moves into the path of the ultrasound beam. One pearl is to move the probe to the patient's right while simultaneously aiming the probe toward the patient's left shoulder, to use more of the fluid-filled liver as an acoustic window. Having the patient take a deep inspiration may also improve imaging by moving the heart down toward the probe.

Finally, patients with abdominal pain may not be able to tolerate this examination, although bending the knees may be helpful. One may need to image the heart from another window if these tips do not resolve such problems.

Apical Window
Patient position For the apical view, first roll the patient into the left lateral decubitus position to bring the heart closer to the lateral chest wall.

Probe position Feel for the point of maximal impulse on the lateral chest wall and then place the transducer at this point, which will generally be just below the nipple line in men and under the breast in women. For the apical view, the probe marker will be oriented toward the patient's right elbow (**Fig. 15**).

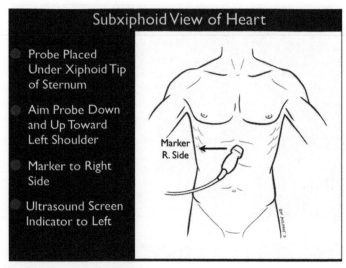

Fig. 13. Subxiphoid view: probe position.

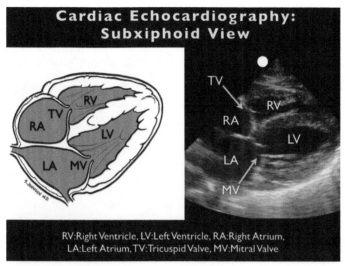

Fig. 14. Subxiphoid view: anatomy.

Anatomic and sonographic correlation The apical window allows for detailed assessment of the relative sizes and movements of all 4 cardiac chambers in relation to one another (**Fig. 16**). This view, like the subxiphoid window, images the right side of the heart well.

The first standard view from this window is the apical 4-chamber view (**Fig. 17**). From this position, the probe can then be angled more superiorly to obtain the apical 5-chamber view (**Fig. 18**), which includes the aortic valve and proximal aorta, the "fifth chamber," identified in the center of the image. The apical 2-chamber view is another variant, whereby the probe is moved laterally on the chest wall to focus the image on the left side of the heart. For Doppler assessment of the mitral, tricuspid, and aortic valves, the apical window is optimal (**Fig. 19**).

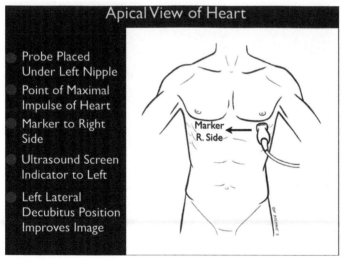

Fig. 15. Apical view: probe position.

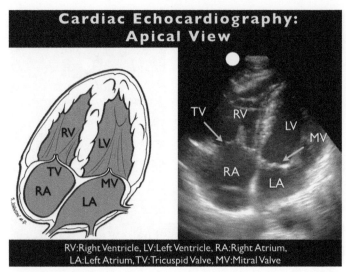

Fig. 16. Apical view: anatomy.

Imaging tips and tricks From the starting probe position at the point of maximal impulse on the chest wall, one can then adjust the probe position on the chest wall to obtain an optimal view. The probe can be moved slightly vertically, up or down, or horizontally, medially or lateral, until the best 4-chamber apical image comes into view.

Orient the probe so that the 4-chamber view includes both the mitral and tricuspid valves. This action confirms that both the left and right chambers are seen in the widest dimensions and avoids slicing tangentially through the heart. The probe may need to be aimed slightly more medially to achieve this view. Obtaining the widest chamber view is critical to obtaining correct measurements and for the assessment of right heart strain (see later discussion).

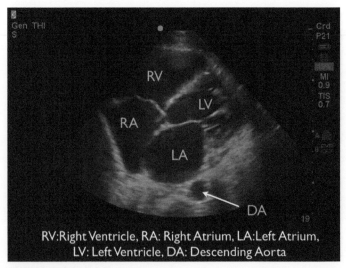

Fig. 17. Apical 4-chamber view.

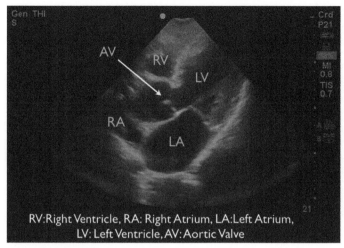

RV:Right Ventricle, RA: Right Atrium, LA:Left Atrium,
LV: Left Ventricle, AV: Aortic Valve

Fig. 18. Apical 5-chamber view.

Other less used cardiac views
Suprasternal notch view This view is used to assess the aortic arch, and is obtained by placing the transducer into the suprasternal area just superior to the sternal notch, with the indicator oriented toward the patient's right (**Fig. 20**).

This view may be difficult in a patient with a relatively high body mass index, as the probe must first fit into this notch and then be angled inferiorly to aim into the chest. Occasionally, abnormality of the aortic arch (aneurysm, dissection) can be identified from this view (**Fig. 21**).

Evaluation of the inferior vena cava
Patient position Position the patient in the supine position for this examination.

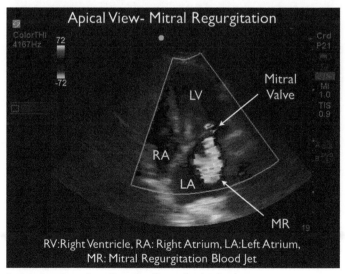

RV:Right Ventricle, RA: Right Atrium, LA:Left Atrium,
MR: Mitral Regurgitation Blood Jet

Fig. 19. Apical 4-chamber view: Doppler flow of mitral valve.

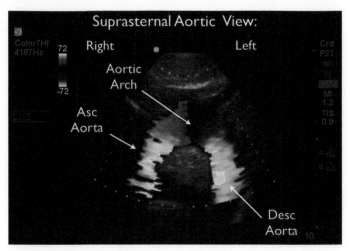

Fig. 20. Suprasternal view: normal.

Probe position From the subxiphoid window, there are several variant views that can be used to image the IVC. First identify the right atrium in the 4-chamber subxiphoid view. Then rotate the probe more inferiorly toward the spine, to visualize the IVC as it runs from the right atrium through the liver to join with the 3 hepatic veins. Next, swivel the probe from the subxiphoid 4-chamber view to the subxiphoid 2-chamber view, by moving the probe to a vertical orientation with the indicator oriented superiorly. This action allows for imaging of the right ventricle above the left ventricle. The aorta typically comes into view in a long-axis orientation seen inferior to the heart (**Fig. 22**). From this plane, moving the probe toward the patient's right side will then bring the IVC into view (**Fig. 23**).

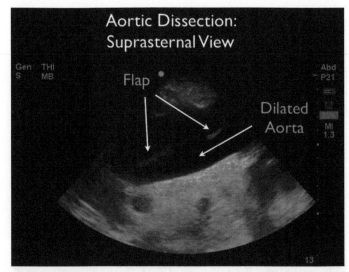

Fig. 21. Suprasternal view: aortic dissection. (*Courtesy of* Diku Mandavia, MD, Department of Emergency Medicine, Los Angeles County + USC Medical Center, Los Angeles, CA.)

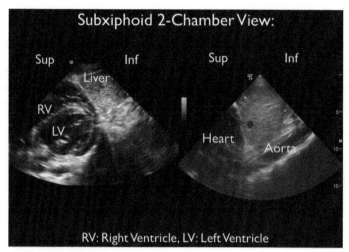

Fig. 22. Subxiphoid 2-chamber view: aorta, long axis.

Anatomic and sonographic correlation Current recommendations for the measurement of the IVC are at the point just inferior to the confluence with the hepatic veins, approximately 2 cm from the junction of right atrium and IVC.[19] Examining the IVC in short axis, as a circular structure, is recommended as the first step. This view potentially avoids a falsely low measurement that can occur through evaluation from the long-axis plane by slicing off to the side of the vessel, a pitfall known as the cylinder tangent effect. The probe can then be turned to image the IVC in the long-axis plane, to further confirm the accuracy of vessel measurements (see later discussion).

Imaging tips and tricks Occasionally, the aorta and the IVC may be confused with one another. The aorta can be identified as a thicker-walled and pulsatile structure with more prominent branch vessels. By contrast, the IVC has thinner walls, is often

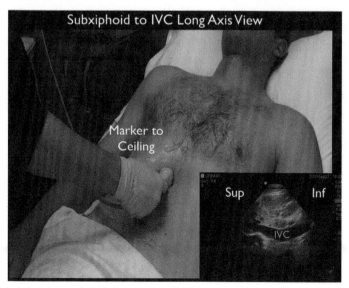

Fig. 23. Subxiphoid view: inferior vena cava (IVC).

compressible with the probe, and can be seen to move through the liver. Although the IVC may have pulsations owing to its proximity to the aorta, color Doppler ultrasonography will further discriminate the arterial pulsations of the aorta from the respiratory phasic movement of blood in the IVC (**Figs. 24** and **25**).

A gas-filled stomach may obscure the view of the IVC from the subxiphoid position. In this situation, the IVC may be evaluated in a long-axis orientation from a lateral, mid-axillary or anterior-axillary view, by using the liver as an acoustic window. The probe is placed on the superior aspect of the right lateral abdomen (similar to a more midsagittal right upper quadrant FAST position) and aimed above the kidney, to image the IVC and aorta (**Fig. 26**).[20]

CARDIAC ABNORMALITY DETECTABLE ON BEDSIDE ULTRASONOGRAPHY
Case 1

A 64-year-old woman with a history of breast cancer presents to the emergency department (ED) with acute shortness of breath and chest pain. She states that the disease has been "in remission" and that she has not received chemotherapy in the past 3 years. She appears acutely ill with the following vital signs: blood pressure 74/58 mm Hg, heart rate 120 beats/min, respiratory rate 30 breaths/min, temperature 36.7 C (98 F), and pulse oximetry 94% on room air. Rales are auscultated in both lungs, but it is difficult to hear heart tones. An electrocardiogram (EKG) reveals a low voltage tracing, without ischemic changes. Portable chest radiography demonstrates an enlarged cardiac silhouette and scattered lung opacities. Focused echocardiography is performed immediately, and an image is taken from the subxiphoid 4-chamber view (**Fig. 27**).

Diagnosis of Pericardial Effusions and Cardiac Tamponade

Pathophysiology
The image taken from this patient demonstrates a circumferential pericardial effusion with evidence of tamponade physiology, visualized as diastolic compression of the right ventricle. Published studies have documented that pericardial effusions may be encountered relatively commonly in critical patients with acute shortness of breath, respiratory failure, shock, and cardiac arrest.[21,22] Fortunately, the literature also suggests that EPs with focused echocardiographic training can accurately identify effusions.[23]

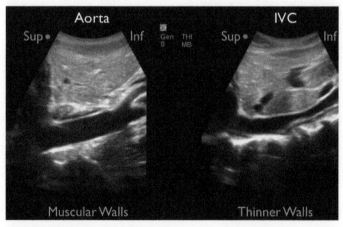

Fig. 24. Long-axis view: aorta and IVC.

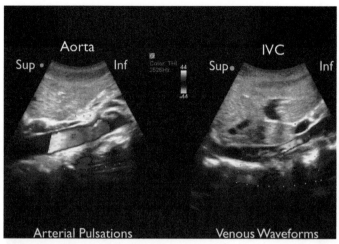

Fig. 25. Color-flow Doppler: IVC and aorta.

Pericardial effusions can result in hemodynamic instability as the pressure in the thick and fibrinous pericardial sac acutely increases, resulting in reduced cardiac filling.[24] Acute pericardial effusions as small as 50 mL may result in tamponade, an important fact to remember in managing the trauma patient. Conversely, in chronic conditions, the pericardium may slowly stretch to accommodate large effusions over time without resulting in tamponade physiology.[25]

Sonographic appearance of pericardial effusions
Pericardial effusions are generally recognized by a black, or anechoic, appearance on ultrasonography. However, effusions that result from an inflammatory or infectious condition may have a lighter gray, or more echogenic, appearance. In addition, as blood clots, traumatic pericardial effusions will take on a more hyperechoic appearance (**Fig. 28**).

Grading scale for the size of pericardial effusions
One scale for determining the size of the effusion is shown in **Table 6**.[11]

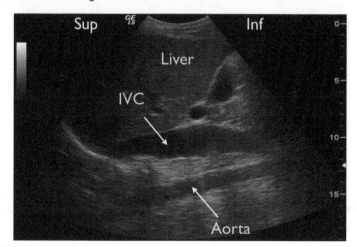

Fig. 26. Right lateral hepatic view, long axis orientation: IVC and aorta.

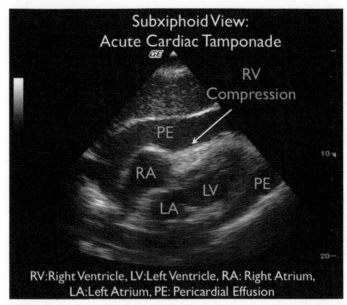

Fig. 27. Subxiphoid view: cardiac tamponade.

Specific echocardiographic windows for the diagnosis of pericardial effusions
Parasternal long-axis view

Location of effusions From this view with the patient recumbent, smaller effusions will first layer posteriorly behind the heart. As effusions grow in size, they will surround the heart in a circumferential manner and will move into the anterior pericardial space.[25] Most effusions will be free flowing in the pericardial sac, although occasionally loculated effusions may occur. These effusions typically occur in patients who have undergone cardiac surgery and in inflammatory conditions.[26]

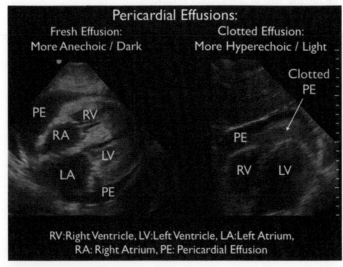

Fig. 28. Types of pericardial effusions.

Table 6
Grading scale for pericardial effusions

A. Small:
    Less than 1 cm depth, noncircumferential around heart
B. Moderate:
    Less than 1 cm depth, circumferential around heart
C. Large:
    More than 1 cm depth, circumferential around the heart

The critical landmarks for detection of a pericardial effusion from this view are the descending aorta and the posterior pericardial reflection. The descending aorta will appear as a cylinder directly behind the left atrium, in the area just posterior to the mitral valve. The posterior pericardial reflection will be identified as a hyperechoic or bright structure, immediately anterior to the descending aorta. Select the appropriate depth of the sonographic image so that the descending aorta and pericardial reflection are identified posteriorly on the screen.

Differentiation of pleural from pericardial fluid These landmarks are key to the diagnosis of a pericardial effusion and differentiation from a left pleural effusion. Pericardial effusions will be located anterior to the descending aorta and above the posterior pericardial reflection. By contrast, pleural effusions will be located posterior to the descending aorta and below the posterior pericardial reflection (**Figs. 29–31**). To further confirm the presence of a left pleural effusion, the probe may be moved to a lateral position on the chest wall and aimed above the diaphragm to visualize the lower thoracic cavity (Please refer to the Thoracic Ultrasound article by Lobo and colleagues elsewhere in this issue).

Pericardial fat pad A pericardial, or epicardial, fat pad may at times be confused with a pericardial effusion. The typical location for this structure is in the area just anterior to the heart and below the anterior, or near-field, pericardial reflection, lying within the pericardial sac. The fat pad often has a classic appearance, with an interspersed speckling of bright, or hyperechoic, regions.

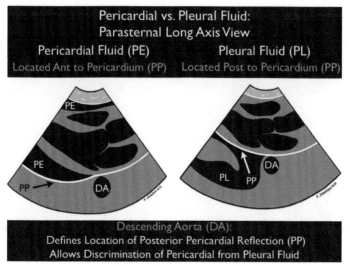

Fig. 29. Parasternal long-axis view: pericardial versus pleural fluid.

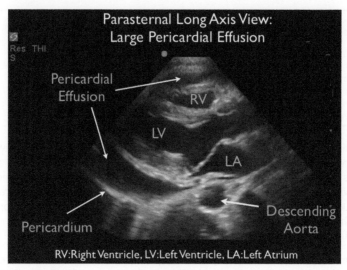

Fig. 30. Pericardial fluid.

From the parasternal view, an isolated anterior location is more suggestive of a fat pad, and not an effusion. For an effusion to be visualized only in the anterior aspect of the pericardial sac, a circumferential effusion would usually be present. This is the case with the great majority of free flowing effusions. In these patients, an isolated 'echo-dense' structure, without an associated posterior effusion, is more likely to be a pericardial, or epicardial, fat pad. A rare exception to this general rule is the loculated pericardial effusion, which may accumulate anteriorly. However, this is seen more commonly in post-cardiac surgery patients or in inflammatory pericardial conditions.

From the subxiphoid view, the pericardial, or epicardial, fat pad would be seen closer to the probe, anterior to the heart and below the inferior, or near-field, pericardial reflection, lying within the pericardial sac (**Fig. 32**).

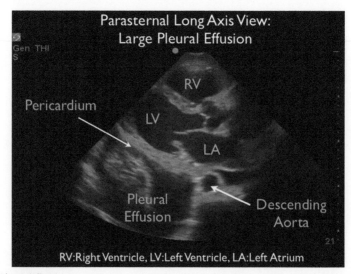

Fig. 31. Pleural fluid.

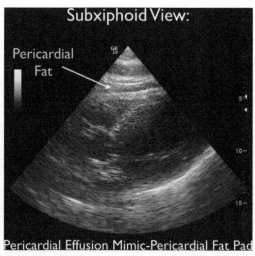

Fig. 32. Pericardial fat pad.

Subxiphoid view

Location of effusions To identify a pericardial effusion from this view, the depth of the image should be set so as to adequately view the entire heart and the pericardium, including both the near-field and far-field pericardial reflections (**Fig. 33**). Because the subxiphoid window is taken from a position inferior to the heart, small effusions will typically layer out with gravity along the near-field, or inferior, pericardial reflection. This is noted most prominently in cases where the patient has been in an upright position prior to the exam. Larger effusions will spread to surround the heart circumferentially.

Differentiation of pericardial effusion from ascites One pitfall of the subxiphoid view is that ascites may at times be confused with a pericardial effusion. Differentiation

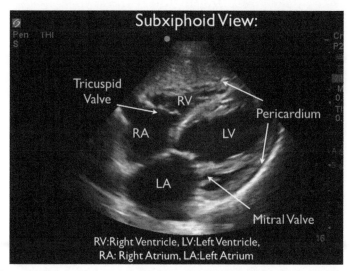

Fig. 33. Normal subxiphoid view: inferior (near-field) pericardial reflection at the top of the image and superior (far-field) pericardial reflection at the bottom.

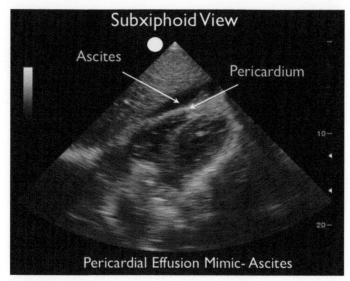

Fig. 34. Subxiphoid view: ascites.

between the two is possible by noting that ascites will be located closer to the probe, surrounding the liver within the abdominal cavity and outside the pericardial sac, as indicated by a position above the near-field pericardial reflection (**Fig. 34**). In contrast, a pericardial effusion will be located within the pericardial sac, below the near-field pericardial reflection and adjacent to the heart (**Fig. 35**).

Apical view Pericardial effusions can be well visualized from this window (**Fig. 36**).

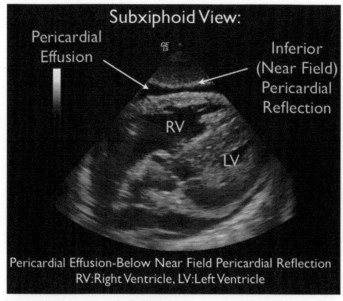

Fig. 35. Subxiphoid view: pericardial effusion.

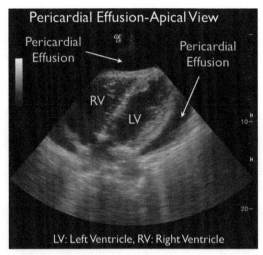

Fig. 36. Apical view: pericardial effusion.

Echocardiographic diagnosis of cardiac tamponade

Defining ultrasonography findings When pericardial effusions accumulate and the pressure in the pericardial sac rises, the lower-pressure circuit of the right heart is affected first, best recognized as an inability of these chambers to fully expand during the relaxation phase of the cardiac cycle. Cardiac tamponade is thus classically defined on ultrasonography as diastolic collapse of either the right atrium or the right ventricle (**Figs. 37** and **38**). The subxiphoid and apical windows are usually best for this evaluation.

Although both right heart chambers should be evaluated, diastolic collapse of the right ventricle is a more specific finding. The right atrium may take on an appearance of a "furiously contracting chamber" with hyperdynamic atrial contractions and exaggerated movements as tamponade progresses (**Fig. 39**), and this can make separation of systolic contraction from diastolic collapse more difficult.

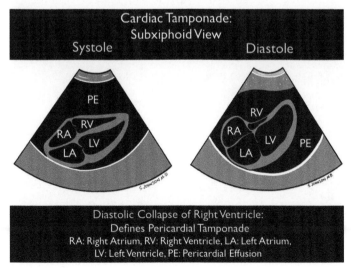

Fig. 37. Subxiphoid view: tamponade.

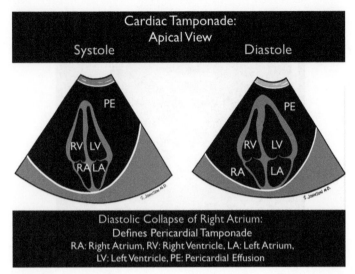

Fig. 38. Apical view: tamponade.

Diastolic collapse of the right ventricle in tamponade is best understood as a spectrum of sonographic findings from a subtle serpentine deflection of the wall in diastole to complete chamber compression.[27] One pitfall of this general diagnostic strategy is seen in the patient with pulmonary hypertension, in whom diastolic collapse of the right heart may be a very late finding.

Strategies to document tamponade There are several strategies to best document diastolic compression of the right heart in tamponade.[28] The first is to attach an EKG monitoring lead to the ultrasound machine to allow for simultaneous display with the echocardiogram and determination of cardiac phases. M-mode ultrasonography can also be used to assess for collapse of the diastolic chamber. From the

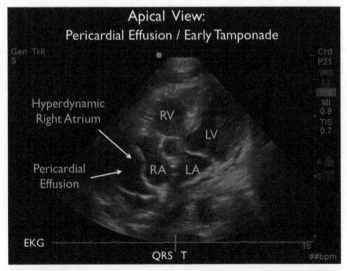

Fig. 39. Cardiac tamponade: right atrial collapse. EKG, electrocardiogram; LA, left atrium; LV, left ventricle; RA, right atrium; RV, right ventricle.

parasternal long-axis view, the cursor is oriented so that it simultaneously crosses both the right ventricular outer wall and the anterior leaflet of the mitral valve. Diastole would be recognized as the period of the opening of the mitral valve and concurrent expansion of the right ventricle (**Fig. 40**). Paradoxical right ventricular wall inward deflection in diastole would suggest tamponade. Evaluation of the IVC may also be performed to confirm tamponade physiology. A plethoric IVC without respiratory collapse implies tamponade physiology.[29]

A more advanced examination using Doppler ultrasonography allows for one of the most sensitive tests to evaluate for tamponade. From the apical 4-chamber view, color-flow Doppler can first be used to identify the flow of blood through the tricuspid and mitral valves. Pulsed-wave Doppler can then be directed onto the jet of blood through either valve to identify augmented differences in the velocity of flow during the respiratory cycle. An increase in blood flow velocity with inspiration across the tricuspid valve (defined as greater than 25% flow variation) suggests cardiac tamponade physiology (**Fig. 41**). Conversely, a decrease in flow velocity with inspiration across the mitral valve (defined as a change between the respiratory phases greater than 15%) may also be seen in tamponade.[30]

Ultrasound guidance of pericardiocentesis
Although most EPs and CCPs have classically been taught the subxiphoid approach for pericardiocentesis, an extensive review from the Mayo Clinic that looked at 1127 pericardiocentesis procedures found that the optimal position for placement of the needle was the apical position in 80% of patients.[31] The subxiphoid approach was only chosen in 20% of these procedures, because of the interposition of the liver. Ultrasound allows for accurate guidance of the pericardiocentesis needle and guide wire into the pericardial sac (**Fig. 42**). Agitated saline can be used as a form of contrast to confirm needle placement in the pericardial space.[32,33]

Case 2

A 72-year-old man presents to the ED for evaluation of chest pain, cough, and generalized weakness. On physical examination, his vital signs include: blood pressure of

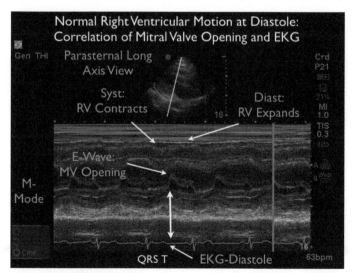

Fig. 40. M-mode correlation with electrocardiogram (EKG): evaluation of right ventricular movement. MV, mitral valve; RV, right ventricle.

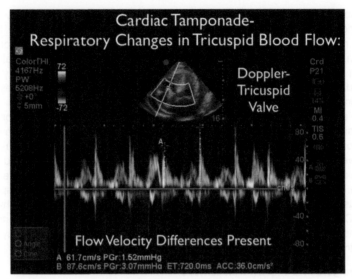

Fig. 41. Tricuspid flow: augmented respiratory variation in tamponade.

78/60 mm Hg, heart rate 116 beats/min, respiratory rate 24 breaths/min, temperature 38.3 C (101 F), and pulse oximetry 92% on room air. He is diaphoretic and ill appearing. The pulmonary examination reveals rales at both bases, and a portable chest radiograph demonstrates bilateral pulmonary infiltrates. Based on this evaluation he is diagnosed with septic shock from pneumonia, and resuscitation is initiated. The relevant clinical questions are first, how good is his cardiac function, and second, what is his volume status? How much fluid should be given to the patient before starting vasopressor agents?

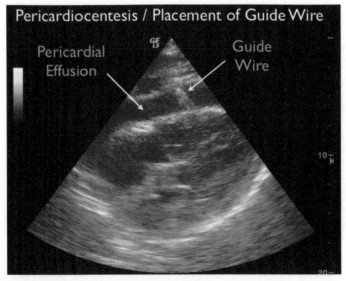

Fig. 42. Ultrasound guidance for pericardiocentesis.

Assessment of Cardiac Contractility

Background
This evaluation incorporates elements of the resuscitation ultrasound protocol written by one of the investigators, known as the RUSH examination (Rapid Ultrasound in SHock in the Critically Ill).[34–36] The first part of this examination is evaluation of the "pump," or assessment for left ventricular contractility. This aspect is crucial, as a relatively high percentage of patients may have a cardiac component to their shock state.[37] Furthermore, published studies have demonstrated that EPs with focused training can accurately evaluate left ventricular contractility.[38]

Grading scale for left ventricular contractility
The examination focuses on evaluating motion of the left ventricular walls by a visual estimation of the volume change from diastole to systole.[39] A ventricle that has good contractility will have a large volume change between the 2 cycles, whereas a poorly contracting heart will have a small percentage change (**Figs. 43** and **44**). The poorly contracting heart may also be dilated in size. Based on these assessments, a patient's contractility can be broadly categorized as being normal, mild to moderately decreased, or severely decreased. A fourth category, known as hyperdynamic, demonstrates small chambers and vigorous, hyperkinetic contractions with the endocardial walls almost touching during systole, often seen as a compensatory response in distributive shock or hypovolemic states.

Evaluation of diastolic heart failure
Although the aforementioned measurements apply to the category of decreased left ventricular contractility as seen in systolic dysfunction, today increasing numbers of patients are being diagnosed with diastolic heart failure. This condition is more commonly seen in patients with chronic hypertension, leading to left ventricular hypertrophy, which may be seen on ultrasonography. It may also be seen in acute conditions, such as pulmonary edema and sepsis.[40,41] The echocardiographic means for detection of this condition involve using Doppler ultrasonography to look for differences in the wave forms (E′ and A′ waves) across the mitral valve, thus allowing for evaluation of decreased left ventricular compliance.[42] However, this is a complex assessment, as the waveforms change during distinct stages of diastolic failure.

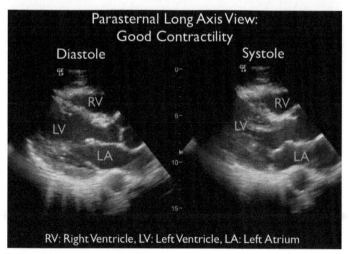

Fig. 43. Left ventricle, good contractility.

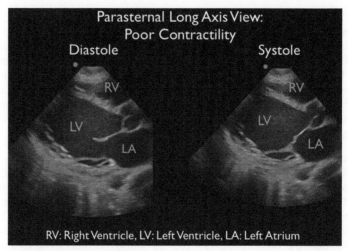

Fig. 44. Left ventricle, poor contractility.

Semiquantitative means for assessment of contractility-fractional shortening
M-mode ultrasonography can be used to graphically depict the movements of the left ventricular walls through the cardiac cycle. The M-mode cursor is placed across the left ventricle just beyond the tips of the mitral valve leaflets. The resulting tracing allows a 2-dimensional measurement of the chamber diameters through the cardiac cycle.

Fractional shortening is calculated according to the following formula:

$$(EDD - ESD)/EDD \times 100$$

where ESD is end-systolic diameter, measured at the smallest dimension between the ventricular walls, and EDD is the end-diastolic diameter where the distance is greatest (**Figs. 45** and **46**).

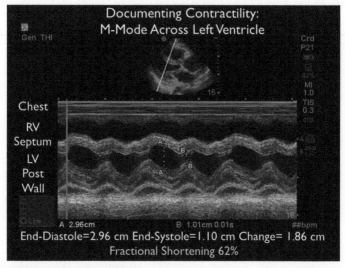

Fig. 45. M-mode, good contractility.

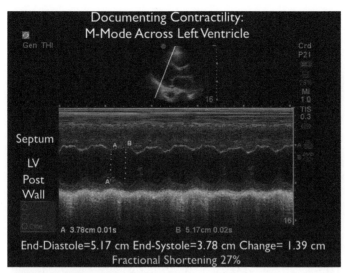

Fig. 46. M-mode, poor contractility.

In general, fractional shortening greater than 30% to 45% equates to a normal ejection fraction.[43] In comparison with the comprehensive and time-intensive volumetric assessment required for measuring ejection fraction, fractional shortening is a semiquantitative method for determining systolic function that is relatively rapid and easy to perform.[44]

Semiquantitative means for assessment of contractility: the E-point septal separation
Motion of the anterior leaflet of the mitral valve can also be used to assess left ventricular contractility. In a normal contractile state, the anterior mitral leaflet as seen from the parasternal long-axis view can be observed to flip open against the septal wall during diastole. As left ventricular contractility decreases, the distance between the fully open mitral valve and the septum correspondingly increases. M-mode is used to measure the degree of mitral valve opening, known as the E-point septal separation (EPSS).[45] The first waveform noted on M-mode is the E wave and represents passive filling of the left ventricle. To measure the EPSS, the M-mode cursor is placed over the tip of the anterior mitral valve leaflet. A normal EPSS is less than 7 mm, whereas an EPSS greater than 1 cm correlates with decreased contractility and a low ejection fraction (**Fig. 47**).[46,47]

Previous literature has supported use of the EPSS as a surrogate measurement of contractility. However, one recent study demonstrated a negative correlation between EPSS and fractional shortening, indicating that more research may be needed on these assessments of contractility.[48] An important caveat is that EPSS does not reflect systolic dysfunction in the setting of mitral valve abnormalities (stenosis, regurgitation), aortic regurgitation, or extreme left ventricle hypertrophy. Furthermore, the measurement should be taken directly perpendicular to the left ventricle. Otherwise, measurements will be taken off-axis and may inaccurately evaluate the EPSS, a concern noted in the aforementioned study.[48]

Quantitative measurements of left ventricular contractility: ejection fraction
This measurement is the 3-dimensional volumetric assessment of cardiac function that is utilized in the cardiac echocardiography laboratory.

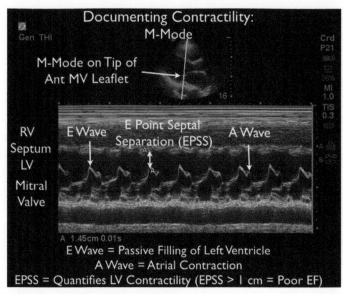

Fig. 47. Mitral valve, E-point septal separation.

Ejection fraction (EF) is defined by the equation:

EF = Stroke Volume/End-Diastolic Volume

This value represents the volume change of the left ventricle during systole. It is best measured by the biplane method of discs, known as Simpson's modified rule, using the concept that the left ventricle represents a bullet-shaped structure.[49] Using this method, the endocardial borders of the left ventricle are traced in 2 orthogonal views during end-diastole and end-systole, generally from the apical 4-chamber and 2-chamber views (**Fig. 48**). Calculation software can then generate the multiple discs representing the left ventricle, and will sum the calculated volumes to provide an accurate ventricular volume. First, the stroke volume is calculated as the difference between the diastolic and systolic volumetric measurements. Next, ejection fraction is calculated using the equation. As this measurement is relatively complex and time intensive, it is not currently a routine part of the goal-directed echocardiography evaluation.

Cardiac index

Measuring cardiac index is another useful advanced echocardiographic application for the assessment of a patient's hemodynamic status, using a combination of B-mode and Doppler measurements.

The cardiac index (CI) is defined as:

CI (L/min per meter squared) = Stroke Volume Index (SVI) × Heart Rate

SVI = Stroke Volume (SV)/Body Surface Area (BSA)

SV (cc) = Left Ventricular Outflow Tract (LVOT) Area × Velocity Time Integral (VTI)

LVOT Area = 0.785 × Aortic valve diameter

VTI = Area Under the Doppler curve, representing the flow of blood passing through the aortic valve with each heart beat.

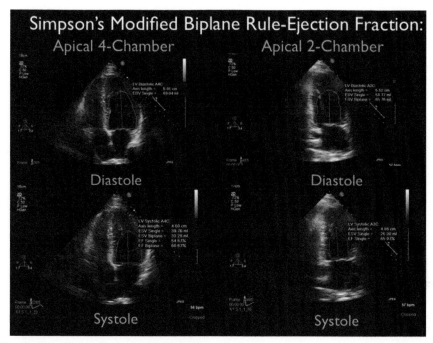

Fig. 48. Simpson method, ejection fraction.

The left ventricular outflow tract (LVOT) diameter is measured from the parasternal long-axis view, taking a measurement between the right aortic cusp and the non-coronary cusp. The velocity time integral (VTI) is an estimation of the distance traveled by a column of blood in 1 systolic beat through the aortic valve.[30,50] The VTI is obtained from the apical 5-chamber view, with the Doppler signal directed at the jet of blood moving out through the aortic valve. The volume of one Doppler pulse is measured by analyzing both the peak velocity and the width of the column, allowing the VTI to be calculated. Multiplying the LVOT area and the VTI together allows for the calculation of the stroke volume (**Fig. 49**). Integrating the body surface area into the equation allows for the determination of the cardiac index. Fortunately, most modern ultrasound machines have the software package necessary to perform these calculations.

A typical cardiac index would be 2.5 to 4 L/min per meter squared. A cardiac index falling below 2.2 L/min per meter squared often indicates a shock state.[51] A recent study demonstrated that the measurement of cardiac output and index can be accurately taken by EP's with limited training.[52]

Evaluation of cardiac contractility in cardiac arrest

In cardiac arrest, the clinician should specifically examine for the presence or absence of cardiac contractions. If contractions are seen, the clinician should look for the coordinated movements of the cardiac valves.[53,54] Specific ultrasonography protocols for use in the setting of cardiac arrest have been used clinically, and further research is ongoing.[55,56] These protocols integrate examination of the heart, the lungs, and the flow in the carotid artery. The subxiphoid view is often used for assessment of the heart during cardiac arrest, as chest compressions can continue with minimal interruption.

If after prolonged advanced cardiac life support resuscitation the bedside echocardiogram demonstrates cardiac standstill, it is unlikely that the adult patient in arrest will

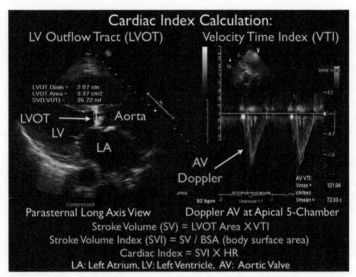

Fig. 49. Cardiac index calculation.

have return of spontaneous circulation.[57–59] The absence of cardiac motion after trauma resuscitation has also been found to be predictive of poor survival rates.[60]

Ultrasonography Evaluation for Volume Status

Evaluation of the inferior vena cava

A noninvasive estimation of the patient's relative intravascular volume can be determined by examining both the relative size and the respiratory dynamics of the IVC. In general, the assessment of the IVC should follow determination of cardiac contractility, allowing the clinician to evaluate both parameters together.

As the patient breathes, the IVC will have a normal pattern of collapse during inspiration, owing to the negative pressure generated within the chest. This respiratory variation can be further augmented by having the patient sniff, or inspire forcefully. M-mode ultrasonography, positioned on the IVC in both short-axis and long-axis planes, can graphically document these dynamic changes in the vessel caliber during the patient's respiratory cycle. Previous studies have demonstrated a positive correlation between the size and percentage change of the IVC with respirations to the central venous pressure (CVP), in an examination termed sonospirometry **(Figs. 50–53)**.[61–69]

Newer published guidelines by the ASE support this general use of the evaluation of IVC size and collapsibility in assessment of CVP, but suggest more specific ranges for the pressure measurements **(Table 7)**.[70]

In intubated patients receiving positive pressure ventilation, the respiratory dynamics of the IVC are reversed. In these patients, the IVC is also less compliant and more distended throughout the respiratory cycle. However, important physiologic data can still be obtained in these patients, as fluid responsiveness has been correlated with an increase in IVC diameter over time.[71]

Evaluation of the internal jugular vein

In the patient in whom a gas-filled stomach or intestine precludes adequate assessment of the IVC, the internal jugular veins may be evaluated as an alternative means of volume assessment. The patient is positioned with the head of the bed elevated to 30°. A high-frequency linear-array probe is recommended for this examination.

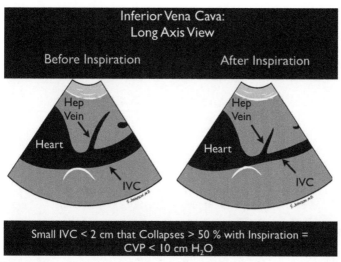

Fig. 50. IVC evaluation of low central venous pressure (CVP).

For volume assessment, one should examine both the relative fullness and the height of the vessel column in the neck using both short-axis and long-axis views (**Figs. 54 and 55**). The percentage change in these parameters with respiratory dynamics should also be evaluated.[72–74]

Case 3

A 72-year-old woman presents for evaluation of acute shortness of breath. She recently underwent right hip surgery and over the last day has become increasingly dyspneic with associated pleuritic chest pain. Her vital signs include: blood pressure 84/62 mm Hg, heart rate 108 beats/min, respiratory rate of 26 breaths/min, temperature 37.2 C (99 F), and pulse oximetry 93% on room air. Her right leg appears larger

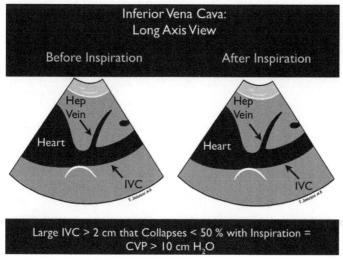

Fig. 51. IVC evaluation of high CVP.

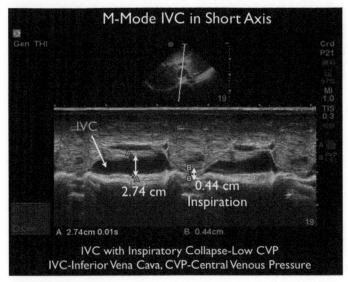

Fig. 52. IVC M-mode: low CVP.

than the left. A chest radiograph shows basilar atelectasis and an EKG demonstrates sinus tachycardia. Bedside ultrasonography is performed and produces the image shown in **Fig. 56**, as taken from the parasternal long-axis view.

Echocardiography for Pulmonary Embolus

Background
Although a CT scan is typically thought of as the current diagnostic standard for pulmonary embolism, focused echocardiography can identify one of the more serious

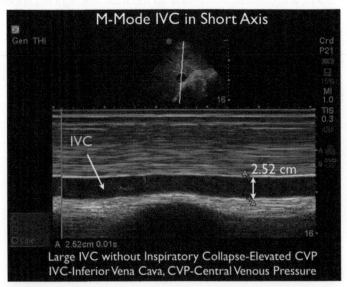

Fig. 53. IVC M-mode: high CVP.

Table 7
IVC and collapsibility
Correlation to Central Venous Pressure (CVP) (ASE Guidelines): A. IVC diameter less than 2.1 cm, collapses greater than 50% with sniff: Correlates to a normal CVP of 3 mm Hg (range 0–5 mm Hg) (while a normal measurement in the healthy patient, this would be considered low in the critically ill patient) B. IVC diameter greater than 2.1 cm, collapses less than 50% with sniff: Correlates to a high CVP of 15 mm Hg (range 10–20 mm Hg) C. Scenarios in which the IVC diameter and collapse do not fit this paradigm: An intermediate value of 8 mm Hg (range 5–10 mm) may be used

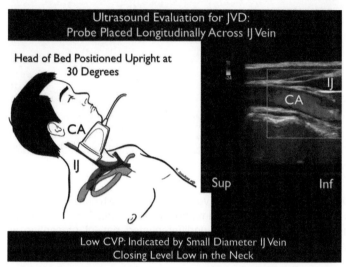

Fig. 54. Internal jugular vein: low CVP.

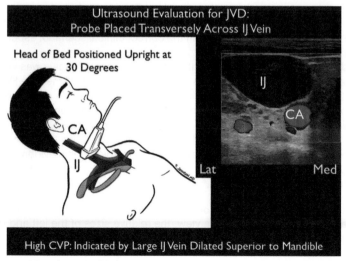

Fig. 55. Internal jugular vein: high CVP.

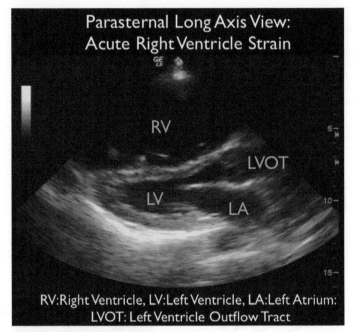

Fig. 56. Acute right ventricular strain.

complications of this disease, right ventricular strain, which correlates with a poorer prognosis and the need for more immediate treatment.[75,76] The examination may also suggest this condition in the undifferentiated patient presenting with shock, potentially leading to a more timely diagnosis.[34–36]

Echocardiography literature for pulmonary embolus

Previous published studies have looked at the use of echocardiography for the evaluation of pulmonary embolus, specifically the presence of right ventricular enlargement caused by acute strain on the chamber. The documented sensitivity of this test is moderate. However, more helpful is the fact that the specificity and positive predictive value of this finding are high in the correct clinical scenario, especially if hypotension is also present.[77–82]

The traditional management of patients with a pulmonary embolus was with anticoagulation alone. More recent guidelines, including one from the American Heart Association in 2011, recommend the combined use of anticoagulants and fibrinolytics in the case of severe pulmonary embolism,[83–86] defined as the presence of acute right heart strain and the clinical signs and symptoms of hypotension, severe shortness of breath, or altered mental status. The most recent literature found that patients with moderate pulmonary embolism may have echocardiographic evidence of pulmonary artery hypertension for some time following the event, further making a case for potential treatment with fibrinolytics.[87]

Echocardiographic findings of pulmonary embolism from cardiac windows

Parasternal long-axis view From this view, the relative sizes of the left and right ventricles can be evaluated. A normal ratio of the right to the left ventricle is defined as 0.6:1, with a greater than 1:1 ratio indicating right ventricular dilatation (see **Fig. 56**).[88,89] Deflection of the interventricular septum toward the left ventricle may also be noted. These sonographic findings confirm the right ventricular strain that may be seen in a severe pulmonary embolus.

In acute right ventricular strain, the chamber will not have the time to compensate by hypertrophy. Typically, a thin wall measuring less than 5 mm will be seen. Acute strain should be differentiated from chronic right heart strain, usually seen in conditions with long-standing pulmonary artery hypertension (such as primary pulmonary hypertension and cases of chronic pulmonary emboli). In chronic conditions, the right ventricular wall will compensate through hypertrophy, often to a size greater than 5 mm. Prominent trabecular architecture of the chamber endocardium and papillary muscles may also be recognized. Faced with the question of whether right ventricular chamber dilatation is acute or chronic, the clinician can use these general rules to decide if more emergent therapy, like fibrinolysis, might be indicated.

Parasternal short-axis view This view also allows for an accurate determination of right ventricular enlargement, and can confirm the findings seen on the parasternal long-axis view. As right ventricular pressures increase, the interventricular septum may be seen to bow from right to left, resulting in a finding known as a "D-shaped chamber" (**Figs. 57** and **58**).[17]

Subxiphoid and apical views Further evaluation of right ventricular dilatation can be made from these views. The apical window is an excellent view for visualization of both right ventricular enlargement and septal bowing. The subxiphoid view can also be used; however, one must take care to aim the probe to capture the widest chamber size and avoid underestimation of dimensions by imaging the right ventricle off-axis.

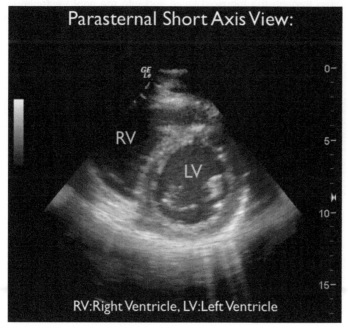

Fig. 57. Parasternal short-axis view: normal.

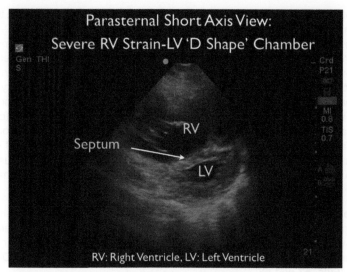

Fig. 58. Parasternal short-axis view: right ventricular strain.

In addition to findings of right ventricular strain, clot may be visualized occasionally within the heart (**Fig. 59**).[90]

Ultrasound Guidance of Transvenous Pacemaker Placement

Guidance of transvenous pacemaker placement can be performed from either the subxiphoid or apical windows. The pacing wire should be observed to pass from the right atrium through the tricuspid valve and into the right ventricle. In the best cases, the wire can be observed to float to a position up against the electrically active

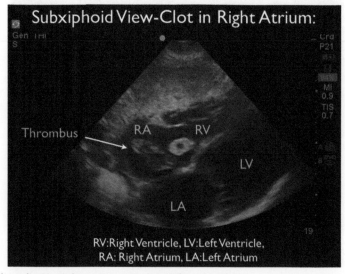

Fig. 59. Thrombus in right atrium entering right ventricle.

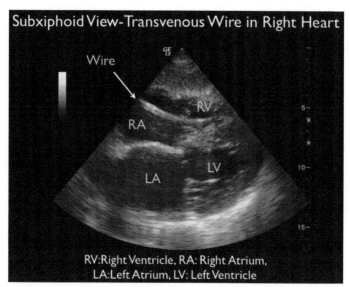

Subxiphoid View-Transvenous Wire in Right Heart

Wire

RA

RV

LV

LA

RV:Right Ventricle, RA: Right Atrium,
LA:Left Atrium, LV: Left Ventricle

Fig. 60. Subxiphoid view: pacer wire present.

right ventricular septum, with mechanical capture confirmed by ultrasonography (**Fig. 60**).

SUMMARY

Today, focused echocardiography allows for the immediate diagnosis of a range of critical pathologic conditions in the patient presenting to the ED or critical care unit with hypotension, shortness of breath, chest pain, or following blunt or penetrating trauma to the chest.[91] Pericardial effusion and cardiac tamponade can be rapidly detected, cardiac contractility and volume status assessed, and the acute right heart enlargement that may indicate a significant pulmonary embolus diagnosed. Using Doppler technology, more advanced echocardiographic evaluations can be carried out, such as assessment for valvular abnormality and hemodynamic monitoring. Cardiac procedures, including pericardiocentesis and placement of a transvenous pacemaker, can be more accurately performed using ultrasonography. For EPs and CCPs caring for the sickest of patients, learning the skill of focused cardiac echocardiography can be of great benefit in providing timely and optimal care.

REFERENCES

1. Moore CL, Copel JA. Current concepts: point of care ultrasonography. N Engl J Med 2011;364:749–57.
2. American College of Emergency Physicians. Emergency ultrasound guidelines. Ann Emerg Med 2009;53:550–70.
3. Akhtar S, Theodoro D, Gaspari R, et al. Resident training in emergency ultrasound: consensus recommendations from the 2008 council of emergency medicine residency directors conference. Acad Emerg Med 2009;16:S32–6.
4. Society for Academic Emergency Medicine. Ultrasound position statement. Available at: http://www.saem.org. Accessed January 20, 2013.

5. Jang TB, Coates WC, Jiu YT. The competency based mandate for emergency bedside sonography and a tale of two residency programs. J Ultrasound Med 2012;31:515–21.

6. Neri L, Storti E, Lichtenstein D. Toward an ultrasound curriculum for critical care. Crit Care Med 2007;35(Suppl 5):S290–304.

7. Bealieu Y. Specific skill set and goals of focused echocardiography for critical care physicians. Crit Care Med 2007;35:S144–9.

8. International Expert Statement on training standards for critical care ultrasonography. Intensive Care Med 2011;37(7):1077–83.

9. Labovitz AJ, Noble VE, Bierig M, et al. Focused cardiac ultrasound in the emergent setting: a consensus statement of the American Society of Echocardiography and the American College of Emergency Physicians. J Am Soc Echocardiogr 2010;23:1225–30.

10. Weekes AJ, Quirke DP. Emergency echocardiography. Emerg Med Clin North Am 2011;29:759–87.

11. Ma OJ, Mateer JR, Blaivas M. Emergency ultrasound. New York: McGraw Hill Publishers; 2008.

12. Cosby KS, Kendall JL. Practical guide to emergency ultrasound. Philadelphia: Lippincott Williams and Wilkins; 2006.

13. Taylor RA, Oliva I, Van Tonder R, et al. Point of care focused cardiac ultrasound for the assessment of thoracic aortic dimensions, dilation and aneurysmal disease. Acad Emerg Med 2012;19:244–7.

14. Fojtik JP, Costantino TG, Dean AJ. The diagnosis of aortic dissection by emergency medicine ultrasound. J Emerg Med 2007;32:191–6.

15. Budhram G, Reardon R. Diagnosis of ascending aortic dissection using emergency department bedside echocardiogram. Acad Emerg Med 2008;15(6):584.

16. Chen RS, Bivens MJ, Grossman SA. Diagnosis and management of valvular heart disease in emergency medicine. Emerg Med Clin North Am 2011;29:801–10.

17. Riley D, Hultgren A, Merino D, et al. Emergency department bedside echocardiographic diagnosis of massive pulmonary embolism with direct visualization of thrombus in the pulmonary artery. Crit Ultrasound J 2011;3(3):155–60.

18. Rozycki GS, Ochsner MG, Schmidt JA, et al. A prospective use of surgeon's performed ultrasound as the primary adjunct modality for injured patient assessment. J Trauma 1995;39:879–85.

19. Wallace DJ, Allison M, Stone MB. Inferior vena cava percentage collapse during respiration is affected by the sampling location: an ultrasound study in healthy volunteers. Acad Emerg Med 2010;17(1):96–9.

20. Howard ZD, Gharahbaghian L, Steele BJ, et al. Midaxillary option for measuring IVC: prospective comparison of the right midaxillary and subxiphoid IVC measurements. Ann Emerg Med 2012;60(4S):S78–9.

21. Blaivas M. Incidence of pericardial effusion in patients presenting to the emergency department with unexplained dyspnea. Acad Emerg Med 2001;8(12):1143–6.

22. Tayal VS, Kline JA. Emergency echocardiography to determine pericardial effusions in patients with PEA and near PEA states. Resuscitation 2003;59:315–8.

23. Mandavia DP, Hoffner RJ, Mahaney K, et al. Bedside echocardiography by emergency physicians. Ann Emerg Med 2001;38:377–82.

24. Grecu L. Cardiac tamponade. Int Anesthesiol Clin 2012;50(2):59–77.

25. Shabetai R. Pericardial effusions: haemodynamic spectrum. Heart 2004;90:255–6.

26. Russo AM, O'Connor WH, Waxman HL. Atypical presentations and echocardiographic findings in patients with cardiac tamponade occurring early and late after cardiac surgery. Chest 1993;104:71–8.
27. Trojanos CA, Porembka DT. Assessment of left ventricular function and hemodynamics with transesophageal echocardiography. Crit Care Clin 1996;12:253–72.
28. Goodman A, Perera P, Mailhot T, et al. The role of bedside ultrasound in the diagnosis of pericardial effusions and cardiac tamponade. J Emerg Trauma Shock 2012;5:72–5.
29. Nabazivadeh SA, Meskshar A. Ultrasonic diagnosis of cardiac tamponade in trauma patients using the collapsibility index of the inferior vena cava. Acad Radiol 2007;14:505–6.
30. Armstrong FA, Ryan T. Feigenbaum's echocardiography. 7th edition. Philadelphia: Lippincott, Williams and Wilkins; 2010.
31. Tsang T, Enriquez-Sarano M, Freeman WK. Consecutive 1127 therapeutic echocardiographically guided pericardiocenteses: clinical profile, practice patterns and outcomes spanning 21 years. Mayo Clin Proc 2002;77:429–36.
32. Salazar M, Mohar D, Bhardwaj R, et al. Use of contrast echocardiography to detect displacement of the needle during pericardiocentesis. Echocardiography 2012;29:E60–1.
33. Ainsworth CD, Salehian O. Echo-guided pericardiocentesis: let the bubbles show the way. Circulation 2011;123:e210–1.
34. Perera P, Mailhot T, Riley D, et al. The RUSH exam: Rapid Ultrasound in SHock in the evaluation of the critically ill. Emerg Med Clin North Am 2010;28:29–56.
35. Perera P, Mailhot T, Riley D, et al. The RUSH exam: Rapid Ultrasound in SHock in the evaluation of the critically ill. Ultrasound Clin 2012;7:255–78.
36. Seif D, Perera P, Mailhot T, et al. Bedside ultrasound in resuscitation and the Rapid Ultrasound in SHock protocol. Crit Care Res Pract 2012;2012:503254 Article ID 503254.
37. Jones AE, Craddock PA, Tayal VS, et al. Diagnostic accuracy of identification of left ventricular function among emergency department patients with nontraumatic symptomatic undifferentiated hypotension. Shock 2005;24:513–7.
38. Moore CL, Rose GA, Tayal VS, et al. Determination of left ventricular function by emergency physician echocardiography of hypotensive patients. Acad Emerg Med 2002;9:186–93.
39. Joseph M, Disney P. Transthoracic echocardiography to identify or exclude cardiac cause of shock. Chest 2004;126:1592–7.
40. Aurigemma GR, Gaasch WH. Diastolic heart failure. N Engl J Med 2004;351:1097–105.
41. Khouri SJ, Maly GT, Suh DD, et al. A practical approach to the echocardiographic evaluation of diastolic function. J Am Soc Echocardiogr 2004;17:290–7.
42. Brown SM, Pittman JE, Hirshberg EL, et al. Diastolic dysfunction and mortality in early sepsis and septic shock: a prospective observational echocardiographic study. Crit Ultrasound J 2012;2:8.
43. Lang RM, Bierig M, Devereux RB, et al. Recommendations for chamber quantification. Eur J Echocardiogr 2006;7(2):79–108.
44. Weekes AJ, Tassone HM, Babcock A, et al. Comparison of serial qualitative and quantitative assessments of caval index and left ventricular systolic function during early fluid resuscitation of hypotensive emergency department patients. Acad Emerg Med 2011;18:912–21.

45. Secko MA, Lazar JM, Salciccioli L, et al. Can junior emergency physicians use E-point septal separation to accurately estimate left ventricular function in acutely dyspneic patients? Acad Emerg Med 2011;18:1223–6.
46. Ahmadpour H, Shah AA, Allen JW. Mitral E point septal separation: a reliable index of left ventricular performance in coronary artery disease. Am Heart J 1983; 106(1):21–8.
47. Silverstein JR, Laffely NH, Rifkin RD. Quantitative estimation of left ventricular ejection fraction from mitral valve E-point to septal separation and comparison to magnetic resonance imaging. Am J Cardiol 2006;97(1):137–40.
48. Weekes AJ, Reddy A, Lewis MR, et al. E-point septal separation compared to fractional shortening measurements of systolic function in emergency department patients. J Ultrasound Med 2012;31:1891–7.
49. St. John Sutton MG, Plappert T, Rahmouni H. Assessment of left ventricular systolic function by echocardiography. Ultrasound Clin 2009;4:167–80.
50. Abraham J, Abraham TP. The role of echocardiography in hemodynamic assessment of heart failure. Ultrasound Clin 2009;4:149–66.
51. Murthi SB, Hess JR, Hess A, et al. Focused rapid echocardiography evaluation versus vascular catheter based assessment of cardiac output and function in critically ill trauma patients. J Trauma 2012;72:1158–64.
52. Dimh VA, Ko SH, Rao R, et al. Measuring cardiac index with a focused cardiac ultrasound examination in the ED. Am J Emerg Med 2012;30:1845–51.
53. Breitkreutz R, Walcher F, Seeger F. Focused echocardiographic evaluation in resuscitation management: concept of an advanced life support conformed algorithm. Crit Care Med 2007;35(5):S150–61.
54. Hernandez C, Shuler K, Hannan H, et al. C.A.U.S.E.: cardiac arrest ultrasound exam. A better approach to managing patients in primary non-arrhythmogenic cardiac arrest. Resuscitation 2008;76:198–206.
55. Breitkreutz R, Price S, Steiger HV, et al. Focused echocardiographic examination in life support and peri-resuscitation of emergency patients: a prospective trial. Resuscitation 2010;81(11):1527–33.
56. Haas M, Allendorfer J, Walcher F, et al. Focused examination of cerebral blood flow in peri-resuscitation: a new advanced life support compliant concept-an extension of the focused echocardiography evaluation in life support examination. Crit Ultrasound J 2010;2:1–12.
57. Blaivas M, Fox JC. Outcome in cardiac arrest patients found to have cardiac standstill on bedside emergency department echocardiogram. Acad Emerg Med 2001;8:616–21.
58. Salen P, Melniker L, Choolijan C, et al. Does the presence or absence of sonographically identified cardiac activity predict resuscitation outcomes of cardiac arrest patients? Am J Emerg Med 2005;23:459–62.
59. Blyth L, Atkinson P, Gadd K, et al. Bedside focused echocardiography as predictor of survival in cardiac arrest: a systematic review. Acad Emerg Med 2012; 19:1119–26.
60. Cureton EL, Yeung LY, Kwan RO, et al. The heart of the matter: utility of ultrasound of cardiac activity during traumatic arrest. J Trauma Acute Care Surg 2012;73:102–10.
61. Kircher BJ, Himelman RB, Schiller NB. Noninvasive estimation of right atrial pressure from the inspiratory collapse of the inferior vena cava. Am J Cardiol 1990;66(4):493–6.
62. Simonson JS, Schiller NB. Sonospirometry: a new method for noninvasive estimation of mean right atrial pressure based on two-dimensional echographic

measurements of the inferior vena cava during measured inspiration. J Am Coll Cardiol 1988;11(3):557–64.

63. Randazzo MR, Snoey ER, Levitt MA, et al. Accuracy of emergency physician assessment of left ventricular ejection fraction and central venous pressure using echocardiography. Acad Emerg Med 2003;10(9):973–7.

64. Jardin F, Vieillard-Baron A. Ultrasonographic examination of the venae cavae. Intensive Care Med 2006;32(2):203–6.

65. Marik PA. Techniques for assessment of intravascular volume in critically ill patients. J Intensive Care Med 2009;24(5):329–37.

66. Blehar DJ, Dickman E, Gaspari R. Identification of congestive heart failure via respiratory variation of inferior vena cava diameter. Am J Emerg Med 2009; 27(1):71–5.

67. Nagdev AD, Merchant RC, Tirado-Gonzalez A, et al. Emergency department bedside ultrasonographic measurement of the caval index for noninvasive determination of low central venous pressure. Ann Emerg Med 2010;55(3):290–5.

68. Schefold JC, Storm C, Bercker S, et al. Inferior vena cava diameter correlates with invasive hemodynamic measures in mechanically ventilated intensive care unit patients with sepsis. J Emerg Med 2010;38(5):632–7.

69. Seif D, Mailhot T, Perera P, et al. Caval sonography in shock: a noninvasive method for evaluating intravascular volume in critically ill patients. J Ultrasound Med 2012; 31:1885–90.

70. Rudski LG, Lai WW, Afilalo J, et al. Guidelines for the echocardiographic assessment of the right heart in adults: a report from the American Society of Echocardiography. J Am Soc Echocardiogr 2010;23(7):685–713.

71. Barbier C, Loubieres Y, Schmit C, et al. Respiratory changes in the inferior vena cava diameter are helpful in predicting fluid responsiveness in ventilated septic patients. Intensive Care Med 2004;30(9):1740–6.

72. Simon MA, Kliner DE, Girod JP, et al. Jugular venous distention on ultrasound: sensitivity and specificity for heart failure in patients with dyspnea. Am J Emerg Med 2011;159:421–7.

73. Jang T, Aubin C, Naunheim R, et al. Ultrasonography of the internal jugular vein in patients with dyspnea without jugular venous distention on physical examination. Ann Emerg Med 2004;44(2):160–8.

74. Jang T, Aubin C, Naunheim R, et al. Jugular venous distention on ultrasound: sensitivity and specificity for heart failure in patients with dyspnea. Ann Emerg Med 2011;29:1198–202.

75. Gifroni S, Olivotto I, Cecchini P, et al. Short term clinical outcome of patients with acute pulmonary embolism, normal blood pressure and echocardiographic right ventricular dysfunction. Circulation 2000;101:2817–22.

76. Becattini C, Agnelli G. Acute pulmonary embolism: risk stratification in the emergency department. Intern Emerg Med 2007;2:119–29.

77. Nazeyrollas D, Metz D, Jolly D, et al. Use of transthoracic Doppler echocardiography combined with clinical and electrographic data to predict acute pulmonary embolism. Eur Heart J 1996;17:779–86.

78. Jardin F, Duborg O, Bourdarias JP. Echocardiographic pattern of acute cor pulmonale. Chest 1997;111:209–17.

79. Jardin F, Dubourg O, Gueret P, et al. Quantitative two dimensional echocardiography in massive pulmonary embolism: emphasis on ventricular interdependence and leftward septal displacement. J Am Coll Cardiol 1987;10:1201–6.

80. Rudoni R, Jackson R. Use of two-dimensional echocardiography for the diagnosis of pulmonary embolus. J Emerg Med 1998;16:5–8.

81. Jackson RE, Rudoni RR, Hauser AM, et al. Prospective evaluation of two- dimensional transthoracic echocardiography in emergency department patients with suspected pulmonary embolism. Acad Emerg Med 2000;7:994–8.

82. Miniati M, Monti S, Pratali L, et al. Value of transthoracic echocardiography in the diagnosis of pulmonary embolism: results of a prospective study in unselected patients. Am J Med 2001;110(7):528–35.

83. Stein J. Opinions regarding the diagnosis and management of venous thromboembolic disease. ACCP Consensus Committee on pulmonary embolism. Chest 1996;109:233–7.

84. Konstantinides S, Geibel A, Heusel G, et al. Heparin plus alteplase compared with heparin alone in patients with submassive pulmonary embolus. N Engl J Med 2002;347:1143–50.

85. Kucher N, Goldhaber SZ. Management of massive pulmonary embolism. Circulation 2005;112:e28–32.

86. Jaff MR, McMurtry S, Archer S, et al. Management of massive and submassive pulmonary embolism, iliofemoral deep venous thrombosis and chronic thromboembolic pulmonary embolism: a scientific statement from the American Heart Association. Circulation 2011;123:1788–830.

87. Sharifi M, Bay C, Skrocki L, et al. Moderate pulmonary embolism treated with thrombolysis (MOPETT trial). J Cardiol 2012;111:273–7.

88. Vieillard-Baron A, Page B, Augarde R, et al. Acute cor pulmonale in massive pulmonary embolism: incidence, echocardiographic pattern, clinical implications and recovery rate. Intensive Care Med 2001;27(9):1481–6.

89. Mookadam F, Jiamsripong P, Goel R, et al. Critical appraisal on the utility of echocardiography in the management of acute pulmonary embolism. Cardiol Rev 2010;18(1):29–37.

90. Madan A, Schwartz C. Echocardiographic visualization of acute pulmonary embolus and thrombolysis in the ED. Am J Emerg Med 2004;22:294–300.

91. Nalin Shah B, Ahmadvazir S, Sihgh Pabla J, et al. The role of transthoracic echocardiography in the evaluation of the patient with acute chest pain. Eur J Emerg Med 2012;19:277–83.

Thoracic Ultrasonography

Viveta Lobo, MD[a],*, Daniel Weingrow, DO[b],
Phillips Perera, MD, RDMS[a], Sarah R. Williams, MD[a],
Laleh Gharahbaghian, MD[a]

KEYWORDS

- Thoracic ultrasound • Lung ultrasound • Emergency ultrasound • Pleural effusion
- Thoracentesis • Pneumothorax • Pulmonary edema • Pneumonia

KEY POINTS

- Thoracic ultrasonography (US) provides a better and faster diagnostic alternative to traditional radiographic techniques in the dyspneic and critically ill patient.
- Traditional resources on bedside US emphasize that the lung is not an organ amenable to US evaluation. Over the last few years, this claim has been shown to be false, and many pulmonary applications have become widely prevalent in clinical use.
- US can be used in the evaluation for pneumothorax, pleural effusions, pulmonary edema, acute respiratory distress syndrome, pneumonia, chronic obstructive pulmonary disease, lung masses, and contusions.
- Using US guidance during a thoracentesis decreases the associated complication rate. In addition, US techniques have been developed to assess for endotracheal placement after intubation attempts.

INTRODUCTION: THORACIC ULTRASONOGRAPHY - ITS HISTORY AND EVOLUTION

In the past, ultrasonography (US) was a relatively neglected aspect of bedside emergency ultrasound (EUS). Due to increased resistance in the passage of sound waves through the air-filled lung, image acquisition and interpretation can be challenging. However, sound waves can easily travel through fluid-filled areas of the chest. Thus, US is more sensitive than chest radiographs for detecting disease such as pleural effusions.[1] In addition, US guidance has been found to offer a dramatic decrease in the complication rate of thoracentesis performed at the bedside.[2]

Funding Sources: None.
Conflict of Interest: V. Lobo, D. Weingrow, S.R. Williams, L. Gharahbaghian: None; P. Perera,
Educational consultant: SonoSite Ultrasound.
[a] Division of Emergency Medicine, Department of Surgery, Stanford University Medical Center, 300 Pasteur Drive Alway M121, Stanford, CA 93405, USA; [b] Department of Emergency Medicine, UCLA Olive View/Ronald Reagan Medical Center, 14445 Olive View Drive, North Annex, Sylmar, CA 91342, USA
* Corresponding author.
E-mail address: vlobo@stanford.edu

Critical care physicians, such as Daniel Lichtenstein and others, subsequently demonstrated that the air-filled lung could successfully be evaluated for specific types of pathology and further developed lung US to expand the previously defined group of applications. In 1995, an important study was published that documented the utility of lung US for the diagnosis of pneumothorax (PTX).[3] After this event, many subsequent studies have shown the effective use of US in the diagnosis of a myriad of lung diseases, including pulmonary edema, pneumonia (PNA), acute respiratory distress syndrome (ARDS), lung masses, and pulmonary contusion.[4,5] Current research has also looked at the use of US in confirming endotracheal tube (ETT) placement following intubation attempts.[6]

CASE PRESENTATION

A 64-year-old woman with a history of hypertension, congestive heart failure (CHF), chronic obstructive pulmonary disease (COPD), and intravenous drug use (IVDU) presented to the emergency department (ED) with severe and sudden dyspnea, which progressed over 15 minutes while at rest. The patient did not have relief after paramedics administered albuterol by nebulizer, high-flow oxygen, aspirin, and nitroglycerin.

On evaluation, the patient was in obvious respiratory distress, in the tripod position, with prominent accessory muscle use. She was able to nod to corroborate the paramedic's history, and denied recent travel or trauma. Her vital signs included blood pressure of 180/100 mm Hg, heart rate of 120 beats per minute, respiratory rate of 32 breaths per minute, temperature of 99°F, and oxygen saturation of 90% on a 100% face mask. She was alert, responsive, and cooperative with treatments. On physical examination, she had jugular venous distension, diffuse wheezes with decreased breath sounds at the right base, tachycardia without murmurs, and bilateral peripheral lower extremity edema.

The differential diagnosis in this patient included CHF exacerbation with flash pulmonary edema, noncardiogenic pulmonary edema, COPD exacerbation, PTX, pericardial effusion with tamponade, pleural effusion, pulmonary embolism, acute myocardial infarction, and PNA. The patient was in a critical status with impending respiratory failure. The correct diagnosis must be made expeditiously and the appropriate treatment rendered immediately to avoid imminent decompensation. Bedside US can allow for a more accurate clinical assessment and provision of targeted therapy to better address the patient's acute condition.

BENEFITS OF THORACIC US

Dyspnea is a common complaint in the ED and is disproportionately involved in higher-acuity patients.[7] The Centers for Disease Control document that more than 3.5 million visits each year are made to US EDs with a chief complaint of dyspnea.[8] Accurate and rapid diagnosis is paramount to making correct treatment and disposition decisions. Dyspneic patients often find it difficult to relate the full details of their history. Furthermore, their physical examination findings often have poor accuracy and interrater reliability.[9] Complicating things further, patients with extreme dyspnea often cannot safely leave the ED for advanced imaging tests. Portable radiographs may be ordered, but often take precious time. Many portable chest radiographs are performed with the patient in the supine position, because of trauma or hypotension, making accurate interpretation more difficult. Mastery of point-of-care bedside US in these dyspneic patients can lead to quick and accurate diagnosis, avoiding treatment delay.[10,11]

US PROBE SELECTION FOR THORACIC APPLICATIONS

Traditionally, lung US was performed with an intermediate frequency US probe at 5 to 7 MHz.[3,12] Because many US systems in use in the ED and intensive care unit (ICU) do not have this probe, more modern sonographic studies emphasize use of either the high-frequency 10-MHz to 13-MHz linear array probe or the 3-MHz to 5-MHz phased-array probe for pulmonary applications.

NORMAL LUNG US ANATOMY

US techniques for assessment of the lung rely on the imaging of the pleural line, which represents the interface of the visceral and parietal pleura of the lung closely opposed to one another. In normal lung, the pleural line is found just deep to the ribs and appears as an echogenic horizontal line that moves back and forth as the patient breathes. It often has a shimmering or twinkling appearance known as lung sliding. The comet-tail artifact is another sonographic finding seen in normal lung (**Fig. 1**). It is formed by reverberation echo, which arises from irregularity of the lung surface.[12] It appears as a vertical echogenic line arising from the pleural line and extending posteriorly down into the lung tissue by a few millimeters (**Fig. 2**). To best visualize this pleural line with its lung sliding and comet-tail artifacts, the high-frequency linear array probe is used. However, the lower-frequency phased-array probe can also visualize this interface, with the depth turned to a more superficial setting.[3,13]

Lichtenstein and Menu[3] showed that lung sliding has a sensitivity of 95.3%, a specificity of 91.1% and a negative predictive value of 100% for excluding PTX when compared with chest radiograph or computed tomography (CT). They found that the significant strength of this technique is that it can immediately rule out anterior pneumothoraces. Lichtenstein and colleagues[12] also found that in a prospective study of 146 hemithoraces, the presence of a comet-tail artifact had a sensitivity of 100% and specificity of 60% for normal lung.

Another normal US finding of the lung is the sonographic A-line. This reverberation artifact results in bright white, hyperechoic semicircular repeating horizontal lines, which are found deep to the pleural line (**Fig. 3**).[14] In contrast to the comet-tail artifact, A-lines do not slide back and forth with respirations. These lines are best visualized with a lower-frequency probe (3–5 MHz).

An additional normal artifact found in lung US is a mirror image of the liver and spleen above the diaphragm. This artifact is best seen in the lateral coronal views of

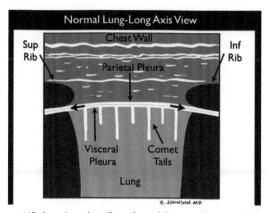

Fig. 1. A normal lung US showing the ribs, pleural line, and comet-tail artifacts.

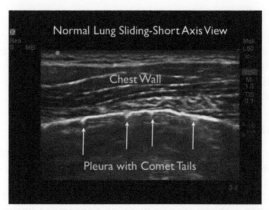

Fig. 2. US of a normal lung showing the hyperechoic pleural line, with comet-tail artifacts.

the lower thoracic cavity using the low-frequency 3-MHz to 5-MHz probe. Because the lung is filled with air, it is difficult to visualize the normal lung parenchyma on US. When an ultrasound is performed from below the diaphragm looking superiorly into the thoracic cavity, the sound waves travel through the spleen or liver and are refracted back to the probe by the interface of the diaphragm and the normal lung. The result is a mirror image of the liver or spleen reproduced superiorly to the diaphragm on the US screen, termed mirror image artifact. Another important normal US finding is that the spine will only be seen inferiorly to the diaphragm and not above, due to the interposition of lung and the resultant poor conduction of sound waves through this air-filled organ (**Fig. 4**).

For a regional anatomic definition of the thoracic cavity, experts have divided the lung into 8 different zones (**Fig. 5**). This distinction can allow for interrogation and proper documentation of specific regions affected by specific disease.[15]

IMAGING FOR PNEUMOTHORAX (PTX)

Patients with PTX may have rapid decompensation, necessitating acute management with placement of a needle or tube thoracostomy. Chest radiographs have served as the traditional diagnostic test for this disease in both medical and trauma patients. However, they have limited sensitivity, because air released from a PTX typically

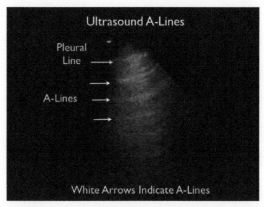

Fig. 3. US A-lines are a horizontal reverberation artifact and a normal lung US finding.

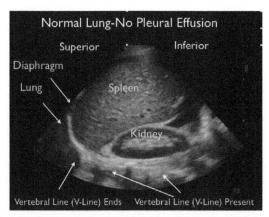

Fig. 4. Normal US of the thoracic cavity. Vertebral line is noted to end above the diaphragm, caused by the presence of intervening lung and lack of fluid.

accumulates in the nondependent anterior-medial and apical aspects of the thoracic cavity, areas that are difficult to evaluate on chest radiography.[16]

Although CT is the gold standard for the diagnosis of PTX, it can be unsafe to transport the critical patient away from the resuscitation area. In addition, higher exposure to radiation is associated with this imaging modality.

Lung US has been found to be sensitive in the detection of PTX in both medical and trauma patients, because it has the ability to evaluate these critical anterior chest areas.[17,18] In a 2010 evidence-based review that included 606 patients,[19] the sensitivity and specificity of supine chest radiographs were 28% to 75% and 100%, respectively. In contrast, the sensitivity and specificity for lung US detection of PTX were 86% to 96% and 97% to 100%, respectively. In a 2012 review on US for PTX,[20] 8 studies with 1048 patients were pooled in the US arm and 7 studies with 864 patients were pooled in the chest radiograph arm. US showed a sensitivity of 90.9%, specificity of 98.2%, positive likelihood ratio of 50.5, and negative likelihood ratio of 0.09. Chest radiography showed a sensitivity of 50.2%, specificity of 99.4%, positive likelihood ratio of 83.7, and negative likelihood ratio of 0.50.

The use of US for the detection of PTX has also been shown to decrease the time to diagnosis, with US requiring an average of 2.3 minutes versus 19.9 minutes for chest

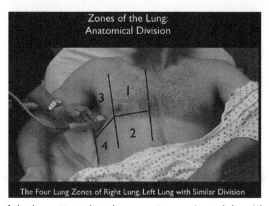

Fig. 5. The zones of the lung. Note that there are 4 zones in each hemithorax, for a total of 8 zones.

radiography.[21] US for PTX has been used accurately in the prehospital setting.[22] Because of this accuracy of US for PTX, the extended focused sonography in trauma (E-FAST) examination incorporates thoracic evaluation for PTX.[23]

Basic US Technique for PTX Detection: Probe Selection and Placement

When evaluating a patient for a PTX, start by using a higher-frequency 10-MHz to 13-MHz linear array probe. The lower-frequency 3-MHz to 5-MHz phased-array probe can be used for this examination, although the images are not so clear. Several presets available on the US machine can be used for this application, but generally a soft tissue setting works best.

In a supine patient, or a patient sitting upright, the probe is placed on the highest position of the anterior chest wall, because air from a PTX rises.[24] This location is often the second or third intercostal space in the midclavicular line (**Fig. 6**). A second position along the lateral chest wall in the mid-axillary line can also be assessed when the clinical suspicion is high for pneumothorax.

Start the scan with the probe oriented so that the indicator is pointing toward the patient's head (**Fig. 7**).

The image should reveal both the superior and inferior ribs, with the hyperechoic pleural line just deep to the ribs (see **Fig. 1**). This sign has been referred to as the bat-wing sign. After obtaining this view, swivel the probe to a short-axis orientation between the ribs to further examine more of the pleural line, without interference of the rib shadows. Care should be taken to avoid mistaking the more superficial rib for the pleural line, because both appear bright or hyperechoic.

Look for normal lung sliding and the presence of comet tails through several respiratory cycles. On the patient's left side, one must be aware that the heart comes up against the chest wall and can interfere with views of the lung. Adjustments of the probe position may be required.

US Findings of PTX

In a PTX, a layer of air splits the inner visceral pleura of the lung from the outer parietal pleura of the thoracic cavity. This accumulation of air between the layers prevents the US beam from detecting normal lung sliding, because the visceral pleura is obscured (**Fig. 8**). This single line, made up of the parietal pleura, does not show horizontal respiratory movements. However, in dyspneic patients with PTX, there may be

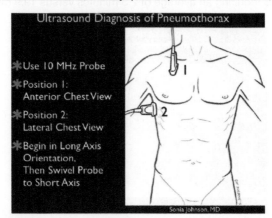

Fig. 6. Probe positions for a PTX scan, anterior chest in the second intercostal space in the midclavicular line, and lateral chest, midaxillary line.

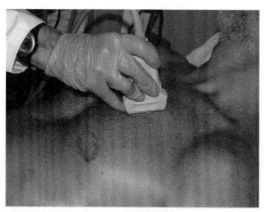

Fig. 7. US probe position for the evaluation of a PTX in the left second intercostal space mid-clavicular line, longitudinal view with the indicator to the head.

exaggerated chest wall movements that cause vertical movements of the parietal pleura, which must be differentiated from horizontal lung sliding. In a PTX, vertical comet tails are also absent. Horizontal repeating lines may instead be noted, because of the reverberation artifact of air.[25] The absence of lung sliding, combined with the lack of the comet-tail artifact, has a specificity of 96.5% for PTX.[12] If there is a question as to the presence of lung sliding and comet tails, the clinician can move the probe to the unaffected hemithorax for comparison, because bilateral PTX are rare.

The Lung Point Sign

Although other US signs are highly sensitive for detecting the absence of PTX, the detection of the lung point sign, or lead point, is a highly specific finding for the presence of a PTX.[26] The lung point is present in an incomplete PTX, when air between the pleural layers interfaces with the normally closely opposed lung pleura. The result is lung sliding in the normal, or unaffected, region of the thorax, with lack of lung sliding in the adjacent region of the PTX (**Figs. 9** and **10**).

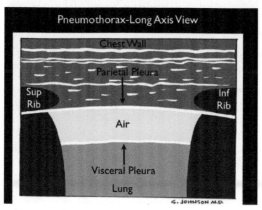

Fig. 8. US evaluation for PTX in longitudinal view showing air separating the parietal pleura from the visceral pleura that inhibits visualization of normal lung sliding.

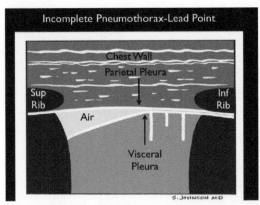

Fig. 9. Lead point of an incomplete PTX showing the transition point, where air accumulates between the 2 pleural layers immediately adjacent to normal lung.

The lung point is best found by evaluating several regions of the chest. In a PTX, air rises and results in a lack of lung sliding on the anterior chest. However, if the PTX is incomplete, part of the lung may still be inflated. This situation is usually discovered in a more lateral position, where air has not yet accumulated (see **Fig. 9**). Therefore, if a PTX is discovered anteriorly, the probe can then be moved to scan sequentially through more lateral and inferior aspects of the chest wall, continuing all the way to the mid-axillary line. One may then be able to find the exact position where the lung in an incomplete PTX slides both up and away from the chest wall. The point at which this occurs is termed the lung point, lead point, or transition point. The presence of the lead point has been shown to have a sensitivity of 66% to 79% and specificity of 100% for PTX.[18,26]

To find the lung point, the short-axis approach is often best. Orient the probe horizontally between the ribs so more of the pleural line can be evaluated. An estimation of the size of PTX can also be approximated by examining for the position of the lead point on the chest wall. A larger PTX displaces more of the lung from the chest wall, resulting in a more lateral position of the lead point. In a complete PTX, the lead point is not encountered on evaluation of either the anterior or lateral chest wall.

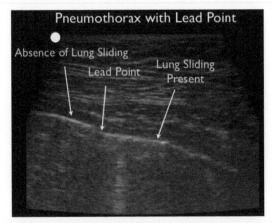

Fig. 10. US of a PTX showing the lead point, the transition between abnormal and normal lung sliding. This is best visualized on real-time B-mode scanning.

M-Mode US for PTX

The presence or absence of lung sliding can be graphically depicted by using M-mode. This technique allows for an assessment of the body's motion in a single vertical plane, as measured over time. A normal lung shows an image with waves on the beach, also known as the seashore sign. Closest to the probe, the chest wall is relatively stationary and demonstrates linear repeating lines (waves), whereas deep to the pleural line, the lung has an irregular and choppy appearance, indicating motion (beach). Conversely in a PTX, the normal lung sliding is lost, and the M-mode evaluation shows only linear repeating horizontal lines. This finding was historically known as the stratosphere sign and more contemporarily termed the barcode sign (**Fig. 11**).[27]

Pitfalls of the PTX US Examination

Because the PTX examination relies on evaluation of the pleural line and lung sliding, there are several conditions that may make the examination unreliable. The first is the presence of extensive subcutaneous emphysema. This situation may make it difficult for the US beam to travel through this subcutaneous air to find the pleural line. The second pitfall is when a pleural effusion or hemothorax has developed together with a PTX. If the amount of effusion or blood is large, fluid may be widely present between the visceral and parietal pleura, effectively prohibiting lung sliding. However, in most cases of small to moderate-sized pleural effusions, the fluid preferentially layers posteriorly. If the probe is positioned on the anterior chest, lung sliding should still be encountered.

The presence of a loculated PTX or large COPD bleb can also make the examination unreliable, because both conditions split the pleural line in defined areas of the lung.[28] A large PNA or lung contusion may further result in a lack of lung sliding, because of pulmonary consolidation. In intubated patients, a right mainstem intubation effectively results in atelectasis of the left lung, resulting in a lack of lung sliding on that side.[29]

IMAGING FOR PLEURAL EFFUSION

Pleural effusions are common manifestations of both pulmonary and systemic diseases. Patients with significant pleural effusions may be in acute respiratory distress and require immediate diagnosis, as well as expedited drainage of the fluid. Although chest radiography has been the reference screening test for pleural effusion, portable

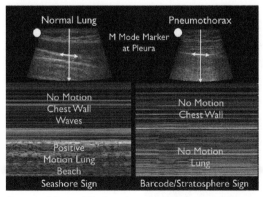

Fig. 11. M-mode of normal lung US showing the seashore sign versus M-mode of PTX showing the barcode or stratosphere sign.

films may miss significant amounts of fluid.[30] Upright and lateral films aid in the detection of smaller effusions. The generally recognized amount of fluid required to blunt the lateral costophrenic angle on an upright posterior-anterior projection is 150 to 200 mL.[31,32] A lateral upright chest radiograph allows detection of as little as 50 mL of fluid.[33] However, in the critical patient, it is often difficult to obtain upright views, much less a lateral film. In contrast to chest radiographs, bedside US has the ability to detect as little as 20 mL of fluid.[33]

One study directly compared chest radiographs with US for the detection of pleural effusion, with CT scan as the gold standard.[34] In this study, chest radiography had a sensitivity of 65%, a specificity of 81%, and a diagnostic accuracy of 69%. US had a sensitivity of 100%, a specificity of 100%, and diagnostic accuracy of 100%. Another study included symptomatically dyspneic patients with pleural effusion, finding a high concordance between US and radiography for the diagnosis of fluid. However, when there was disagreement, US was more accurate than chest radiographs and faster to obtain.[35] Furthermore, US has been shown to have the ability to better quantify the composition of the pleural effusion, as well as determining when complicated or loculated effusions are present.[1]

Patients may also present with dyspnea and have a chest radiograph that shows complete opacification of a hemithorax. This situation can make it difficult to come to an accurate diagnosis, because the differential diagnosis includes both a volume-increasing disease, such as a massive pleural effusion, and a volume-decreasing disease, such as severe atelectasis and consolidation. US has been shown to be helpful in accurately determining the cause of the disorder and in guiding appropriate management.[11,36] Furthermore, evaluation for hemothorax is now a dedicated part of the E-FAST examination, performed as part of the right and left upper quadrant evaluations. Lung US has been shown to be more sensitive and specific for the evaluation of traumatic hemothorax than chest radiographs.[37]

Basic US Technique for Pleural Effusion Evaluation: Probe Selection and Placement

Begin with a lower-frequency 3-MHz to 5-MHz phased-array probe. Elevating the head of the bed (even by a small amount) may cause pleural fluid to accumulate just above the diaphragms, increasing the sensitivity of this examination.

The evaluation for pleural effusion is initially performed from a lateral location on the chest wall, with the probe in a coronal plane, at the midaxillary line, in a subdiaphragmatic location (**Fig. 12**). The probe is angled up to look above the liver, spleen, and the

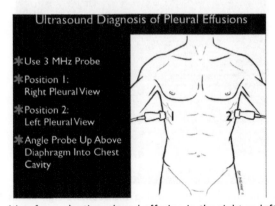

Fig. 12. Probe position for evaluating pleural effusion in the right or left lung.

diaphragms, using the fluid-filled liver and spleen as acoustic windows to the thoracic cavity (**Figs. 13** and **14**). The diaphragms appear as bright hyperechoic lines immediately cephalad to the liver and spleen. In the presence of pleural effusion, there is a dark anechoic space displacing the lung superior to the diaphragm, and the normal mirror image artifact is absent (**Fig. 15**).[27] If a pleural effusion is detected, the clinician can then move the probe sequentially through more superior intercostal spaces to define the full extent of the effusion (**Fig. 16**). Once a fluid collection in the chest is diagnosed, switching to a higher-frequency 10-MHz probe can allow for further characterization of the fluid and definition of the anatomy (**Fig. 17**).

US Findings of Pleural Effusion

With a pleural effusion, the normal mirror image artifact is absent. Instead, there is an anechoic, or black, fluid collection above the diaphragm. Because fluid allows for the improved through-transmission of sound, the spine is seen traversing above the diaphragm when there is a pleural effusion. This finding is known as the V line, or vertebral line, and was recently described in the literature as pathognomonic for a pleural effusion.[38] This sign is a result of a thoracic fluid collection acting as an acoustic window to enable visualization of the posteriorly located vertebral bodies in a line above the diaphragm (**Fig. 18**).

US-GUIDED THORACENTESIS AND THORACOSTOMY

US can be used to guide thoracentesis and tube thoracostomy placement. During a thoracentesis, the pleural effusion can first be examined for septations or loculations, which may suggest a more complicated procedure (**Figs. 19** and **20**). The British Thoracic Society recommends that pleural effusions amenable to safe thoracentesis have at least a 10 mm depth, resulting in sufficient separation of the lung from the outer parietal pleura.[39] The movement of lung should also be viewed over a full respiratory cycle, to examine for intervening lung, which may move into a position located along the planned needle path. The position of the diaphragm should be determined in order to avoid puncturing this structure. In a mechanically ventilated patient, a pleural fluid depth of at least 15 mm, visualized over 3 intercostal spaces, has been shown to be associated with a decreased complication rate.[40]

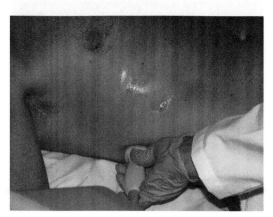

Fig. 13. Right pleural examination, using a 3-MHz probe, with the indicator toward the head and angling upward to evaluate above the diaphragm.

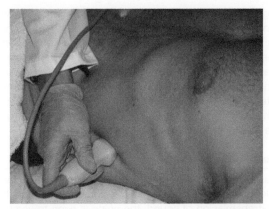

Fig. 14. Probe placed between the ribs to evaluate for a left pleural effusion.

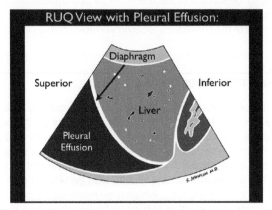

Fig. 15. Pleural effusion on the right upper quadrant view shown above the diaphragm line as anechoic fluid.

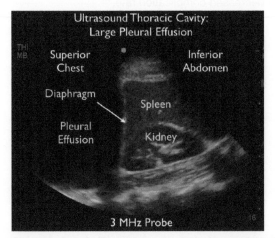

Fig. 16. US image of a large pleural effusion seen above the hyperechoic diaphragm on the right upper quadrant view.

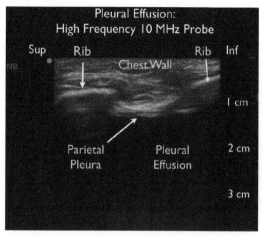

Fig. 17. Pleural effusion noted on the anterior chest wall, using the 13-MHz probe. The effusion appears as anechoic fluid just far field to the parietal pleura.

Basic Technique for Performing US-Guided Thoracentesis

To perform US-guided thoracentesis, a combination of the 3-MHz to 5-MHz and 10-MHz to 13-MHz probes can be used to determine the best position for needle placement. The lower-frequency probe can be used first to obtain a more global view, followed by use of the higher-frequency probe to gain a more detailed view of the anatomy of the area of the planned procedure (**Fig. 21**). Either a static technique, where the patient is positioned and then the optimal needle position marked off and the procedure performed, or a dynamic technique, where the probe is placed in a sterile sheath and the needle is advanced into the effusion under real-time guidance, may be used.

US Confirmation of Tube Thoracostomy Placement

In patients requiring tube thoracostomy, a recent study showed that ultrasound could confirm the appropriate positioning of the chest tube (**Fig. 22**).[41]

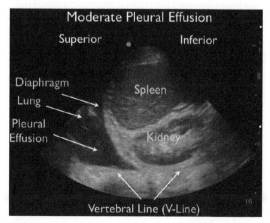

Fig. 18. A moderate pleural effusion on the left upper quadrant view allows for visualization of the vertebral line superior to the diaphragm. Contrast with **Fig. 4**.

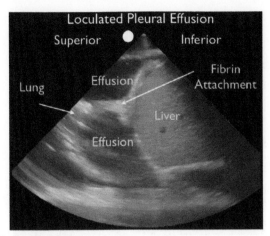

Fig. 19. Loculated pleural effusion.

Literature Supporting US-Guided Thoracentesis

The published data show a definite benefit for the use of US guidance during the thoracentesis procedure to lower the associated complication rate, chiefly that of PTX. A recent literature review[36] combined 23 studies from 1978 to 2010 that evaluated the risk of PTX associated with thoracentesis. The incidence of PTX ranged from 4.3% to 30% of cases without US guidance, and decreased to 0% to 9.1% when US was used. A comprehensive 2010 meta-analysis on this topic[2] pooled 24 studies, which included 6605 thoracentesis procedures. The overall risk of PTX was 6.0%, with 34% of these patients subsequently requiring chest tubes. US guidance for thoracentesis significantly decreased the rate of PTX, with an odds ratio of 0.3. Based on these data, a recent review article urged inclusion of US guidance for thoracentesis as a best-practice guideline, and several medical specialties, including the British Thoracic Society and a panel of international experts, support this position.[39,42]

IMAGING OF PULMONARY EDEMA/CHF

Acute decompensated heart failure is the most common cause of hospital admissions in patients older than 65 years, accounting for greater than 1 million hospitalizations

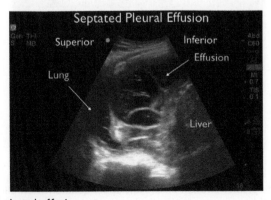

Fig. 20. Septated pleural effusion.

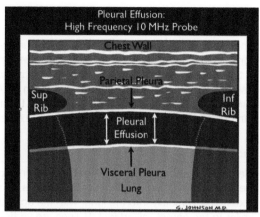

Fig. 21. Pleural effusion seen using a 10-MHz probe that lies between the parietal and visceral pleura.

annually in the United States alone.[43] Chest radiography is relatively specific (76%), but poorly sensitive (67%), for pulmonary edema.[44] The result is that the clinician may have diagnostic uncertainty in diagnosing this condition in up to one-third of patients presenting with acute dyspnea.[45] US techniques used in the evaluation of pulmonary edema include that of the lung, as well as an assessment of cardiac function and volume status.

Pulmonary edema can occur from a variety of causes, the most common being an acute exacerbation of acute CHF. However, noncardiogenic pulmonary edema may be seen as a result of drug, medication, and toxin effects, or high altitude. Physical examination findings (rales, wheezes, extremity edema) may be misleading when considered alone in the diagnosis of pulmonary edema.[46] The multiple causes for this disease all share the common pathway of backup of fluid into the pulmonary vasculature and the interstitial space. US can visualize this interstitial fluid, as well as the pleural effusions that may coexist.

Acute alveolar interstitial syndrome (AIS) is caused by fluid occupying the alveolar spaces. It can be caused by diseases as disparate as ARDS, interstitial PNA, and pulmonary edema. Regardless of the cause, it can be identified with bedside US as having a characteristic appearance.[13]

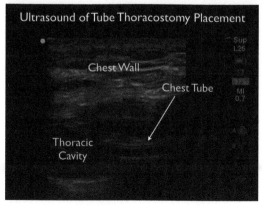

Fig. 22. US of chest tube in thoracic cavity.

Basic Technique for Pulmonary Edema and Alveolar Fluid Evaluation: Probe Selection and Placement

Using the 8 zones of the chest wall (see **Fig. 5**), place the low-frequency 3-MHz to 5-MHz phased-array probe on the chest wall and evaluate each zone using an increased depth setting. Slide and fan the probe through areas within each zone to assess for the characteristic findings described below. Because lung findings, such as A and B-lines are forms of artifact that arise off the pleura, turning off advanced US technology, like tissue harmonic imaging, can coarsen the image and accentuate these lines.

US Findings for Pulmonary Edema and Alveolar Fluid

In patients with alveolar fluid, an artifact known as the US B-line or lung rocket develops (**Fig. 23**). B-lines appear as well-defined bright hyperechoic lines, or rays, arising from the pleural line and extending vertically into the lung, with the appearance of a rocket lifting off in flight. Similar to the comet-tail artifact, B-lines are vertical lines that move with sliding of the lung. However, B-lines are differentiated from comet tails by a deeper penetration of these vertical lines across the image. These lines extend to the far field of the US image without fading out, even with the deeper imaging allowed by the lower frequency 3-MHz probe.[13,47,48]

The development of B-lines results from the thickening of the interlobular septa, because extravascular water or fluid accumulates within the pulmonary interstitial area and alveoli.[46] The B-line pattern has been shown to correlate with pulmonary artery occlusion pressure and resolves after adequate medical treatment of decompensated heart failure has been instituted.[14,49] One recent study reported that B-lines may best be appreciated by positioning the probe in a more lateral, or even in a posterior position. This increased sensitivity of a posterior approach is hypothesized to be a result of the natural movement of fluid with gravity.

When evaluating a patient for AIS, if horizontal A-lines are present and vertical B-lines are absent, interstitial edema is less likely.[50] A positive US study for AIS involves visualizing more than 2 B-lines on the US screen in more than 2 zones of the lung. Some researchers have looked at the number of B-lines per US field across the chest as having a better correlation with the degree of pulmonary edema.[51] Severe pulmonary edema may result in many lung rockets per US field, producing a finding known as lung whiteout (**Fig. 24**). A positive US study for AIS typically seen in pulmonary edema involves

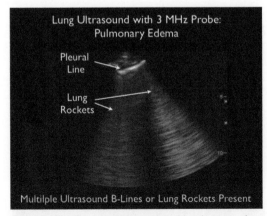

Fig. 23. US B-lines, also known as lung rockets, appear like the rays of a searchlight and arise from the pleural line, extending to the entire far field of the image.

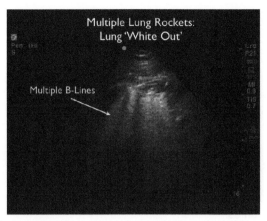

Fig. 24. Multiple lung rockets in severe pulmonary edema appear as a bright echogenic area, often called lung whiteout.

visualizing more than 2 B-lines on the US screen in more than 2 zones of the chest, bilaterally. This finding differs from most cases of PNA, lung contusion and rarer cases of pulmonary edema, in which B-lines may be a unilateral lung finding found in a single or only a few lung zones, indicating a more localized form of AIS.

US EVALUATION OF COPD

As life expectancy increases, COPD and CHF are becoming more prevalent and may coexist in a subset of patients. With sometimes very similar acute presentations, the physician must correctly differentiate between these 2 different pathophysiologic processes. Although there are no definitive US markers for COPD, the A-lines that are seen in normal lung may be more prominent with COPD. Of more help to the clinician is the lack of identifiers suggesting an alternative diagnosis (i.e., B-lines).[52] One study showed that US signs of AIS, noted as US B-lines, were seen in all patients with pulmonary edema, but were absent in most patients with COPD exacerbation (100% sensitivity, 92% specificity).[53] Alternatively, if no B-lines are noted and instead A-lines are seen in the patient with a suggestive history, the diagnosis is more likely to be a COPD exacerbation.

Patients with severe COPD may have large pulmonary blebs, which appear as a lack of lung sliding and may mimic a PTX. However, these blebs may be filled with debris and have a characteristic appearance on US that differs from a PTX (**Fig. 25**).

US EVALUATION OF PNA

PNA comprises both accumulation of alveolar fluid and consolidation within the lung. Although a common diagnosis in the acute care setting, it is not always noted on chest radiographs and may be confused with other disease.[54] However, as lung consolidation progresses, this organ becomes fluid filled and more compact.

Basic US Technique for PNA Assessment

To examine for PNA, use the 3-MHz to 5-MHz phased-array probe to scan through each of the 8 zones of the lung, looking specifically for areas that appear more solid and echogenic and different in appearance from the surrounding tissue (**Fig. 26**).[55]

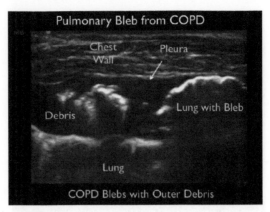

Fig. 25. COPD blebs on US.

A high-frequency probe may also be used to examine for pneumonia, especially if the PNA is believed to be located peripherally (**Fig. 27**).

US Findings in PNA

Several US findings have been established to help identify alveolar consolidation, which takes on the appearance of a liver in the chest in a process termed hepatization.[55–58] Another finding in PNA is the air bronchogram. Air bronchograms represent air-filled bronchi inside the area of lung consolidation and can be seen on US as linear branching and hyperechoic lines within an area of consolidation (See **Fig. 26**).[56,59] In addition, US B-lines or lung rockets may also be seen in areas of the PNA where there is predominant alveolar fluid.[57] In addition, US has a further role in diagnosing complications of PNA, such as a parapneumonic effusion (**Fig. 27**).[60] US can then be used to guide a thoracentesis to confirm the presence of an empyema, before a more definitive drainage procedure.

A thickened pleural line that is unlike the normal thin line of normal lung may be seen in association with pulmonary consolidation. A thick pleural line is seen if the PNA is peripherally located. This finding can also be seen in other conditions like lung scarring, fibrosis, empyema, and pleuritis.

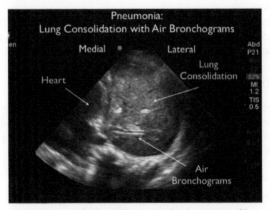

Fig. 26. PNA seen on US using a 3-MHz probe. Note the presence of lung consolidation and air bronchograms.

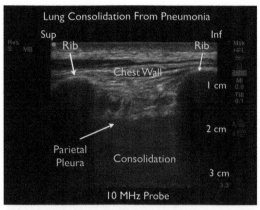

Fig. 27. PNA seen on US using a 10-MHz linear probe.

LUNG MASSES

Lung masses may also be detected on thoracic US.[4] Lung masses are more easily visualized if they are peripherally located close to the pleura or are large. Lung masses appear similar to consolidated lung, taking on the appearance of hepatization with the look of a liver in the chest. M-mode may be used to further discriminate a mass from fluid (**Fig. 28**).

US EVALUATION OF SUCCESSFUL ENDOTRACHEAL INTUBATION

Thoracic US has also been used during endotracheal intubations.[6,61] With US, an esophageal intubation that must be quickly recognized and removed can be easily distinguished. An esophageal intubation has the appearance of 2 discrete round structures within the neck, because the ETT is seen within the esophagus as 1 circular structure posterolaterally to the round, anteriorly located trachea (**Fig. 29**). This structure is best evaluated by placement of the high-frequency linear array probe in a transverse orientation across the neck. If the ETT is correctly positioned within the trachea,

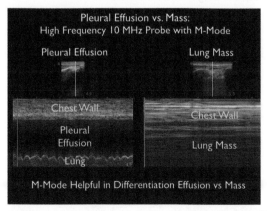

Fig. 28. M-mode scan of a mass shows the anechoic area of the pleural effusion versus echogenicity within a mass.

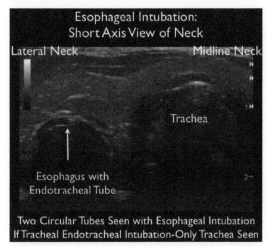

Fig. 29. Esophageal intubation noted as 2 tubular structures in neck. High-frequency probe is placed in the transverse axis across neck. With a tracheal intubation, only the trachea would be seen, making 1 tube apparent on US.

only the single circular structure of the trachea is seen, without an associated tube-filled esophagus located posterolaterally.

US can also be used to confirm successful ETT placement by assessing bilateral lung sliding and evaluating for movement of the diaphragms during ventilation. The lung pulse is a finding associated with right mainstem intubation and represents atelectasis of the left lung.[62] This finding is represented by a characteristic lack of horizontal lung sliding in the left chest. Instead, subtle movements (pulses) of the pleura are seen, which move in a synchronized fashion to the heartbeat (**Fig. 30**). This finding represents the transmission of movement of the heart through the collapsed lung.

To assess for bilateral diaphragmatic movement with successful intubation and ventilation, the 3-MHz to 5-MHz probe can be positioned in the right upper and left upper quadrants and angled above the liver and spleen to detect bilateral, symmetric, diaphragmatic motion with each ventilation attempt. A more recent study specifically examined for motion of the diaphragm from the right subcostal position as a means of identification of adequate lung motion with intubation.[63]

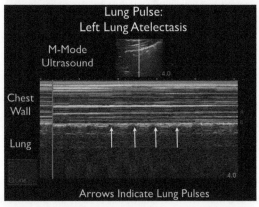

Fig. 30. Lung pulse from right mainstem intubation seen on M-mode.

ROLE OF THORACIC US IN RESUSCITATION OF THE CRITICALLY DYSPNEIC PATIENT

Several resuscitation techniques now emphasize both thoracic and lung US techniques in the resuscitation of the critical patient with acute shortness of breath.[64] These protocols include the BLUE (Bedside Lung Ultrasound in Emergency) protocol and the RADIUS (Rapid Assessment of Dyspnea with Ultrasound) protocol.[65,66] The BLUE protocol focuses on placement of the probe on 3 distinct areas of the chest to diagnose PTX, pulmonary edema, pulmonary consolidation, and effusions. The RADIUS protocol begins with a cardiac evaluation, but then focuses on a pulmonary evaluation looking for similar disease to the BLUE protocol. One recently published resuscitation protocol, termed the FALLS (Fluid Administration Limited by Lung Sonography) protocol, uses lung US techniques to assess a patient's hemodynamic status and to determine fluid needs.[67] The newest US algorithm, the CORE scan, uses bedside US to diagnose common cardiothoracic and vascular causes for decompensation and can be used to guide resuscitation efforts.

CASE DISCUSSION FOLLOW-UP

On arrival to the ED, the patient was noted to be in severe respiratory distress and preparations for intubation were made. A bedside US was performed immediately and showed significant B-lines in 6 of the 8 chest zones bilaterally, associated with small pleural effusions, normal lung sliding, and comet-tail artifacts. Evaluation of the heart showed normal left ventricular contractility, without pericardial effusion or evidence of right heart strain. Electrocardiography did not show any signs of ischemia. Maximal medical therapy was initiated for pulmonary edema and the patient had subsequent dramatic clinical improvement, allowing admission to the floor instead of the ICU. Based on her presentation and clinical findings, the patient was diagnosed with flash noncardiogenic pulmonary edema from heroin use. She was discharged from the hospital 2 days later in good condition.

SUMMARY

Bedside point-of-care thoracic US is a tool that may easily be used to evaluate the critically ill patient presenting with acute dyspnea or shortness of breath, because it can rule in and rule out a wide variety of emergent conditions. As detailed in the case presentation and in this article, US is useful in a wide range of pulmonary disease, including PTX, pleural effusions, pulmonary edema, PNA, lung masses, and COPD. In addition, US has been found to be helpful in the guidance of thoracic and airway procedures. The use of US for thoracic applications is now supported by many research studies and has been incorporated into best-practice guidelines by medical specialties and consensus groups. Bedside thoracic US is a useful tool, which emergency and critical care physicians should consider incorporating into their clinical practice.

REFERENCES

1. Yang PC, Luh KT, Chang DB, et al. Value of sonography in determining the nature of pleural effusion: analysis of 320 cases. AJR Am J Roentgenol 1992; 159(1):29–33.
2. Gordon CE, Feller-Kopman D, Balk EM, et al. Pneumothorax following thoracentesis: a systematic review and meta-analysis. Arch Intern Med 2010;170(4): 332–9.

3. Lichtenstein DA, Menu Y. A bedside ultrasound sign ruling out pneumothorax in the critically ill. Lung sliding. Chest 1995;108(5):1345–8.

4. Koenig SJ, Narasimhan M, Mayo PH. Thoracic ultrasonography for the pulmonary specialist. Chest 2011;140(5):1332–41.

5. Coonar AS, Hughes JA, Walker S, et al. Implementation of real-time ultrasound in a thoracic surgery practice. Ann Thorac Surg 2009;87(5):1577–81.

6. Chou HC, Tseng WP, Wang CH, et al. Tracheal rapid ultrasound exam (T.R.U.E.) for confirming endotracheal tube placement during emergency intubation. Resuscitation 2011;82(10):1279–84.

7. Ruger JP, Lewis LM, Richter CJ. Identifying high-risk patients for triage and resource allocation in the ED. Am J Emerg Med 2007;25(7):794–8.

8. Centers for Disease Control and Prevention. National Hospital Ambulatory Medical Care Survey. NHAMCS-Emergency Department Summary Tables 2010. Available at: http://www.cdc.gov. Accessed September, 2013.

9. Wipf JE, Lipsky BA, Hirschmann JV, et al. Diagnosing pneumonia by physical examination: relevant or relic? Arch Intern Med 1999;159(10):1082–7.

10. Lichtenstein DA, Meziere GA. Relevance of lung ultrasound in the diagnosis of acute respiratory failure: the BLUE protocol. Chest 2008;134(1):117–25.

11. Koeze J, Nijsten MW, Lansink AO, et al. Bedside lung ultrasound in the critically ill patient with pulmonary pathology: different diagnoses with comparable chest X-ray opacification. Crit Ultrasound J 2012;4(1):1.

12. Lichtenstein D, Meziere G, Biderman P, et al. The comet-tail artifact: an ultrasound sign ruling out pneumothorax. Intensive Care Med 1999;25(4):383–8.

13. Lichtenstein D, Meziere G, Biderman P, et al. The comet-tail artifact. An ultrasound sign of alveolar-interstitial syndrome. Am J Respir Crit Care Med 1997;156(5):1640–6.

14. Lichtenstein DA, Meziere GA, Lagoueyte JF, et al. A-lines and B-lines: lung ultrasound as a bedside tool for predicting pulmonary artery occlusion pressure in the critically ill. Chest 2009;136(4):1014–20.

15. Volpicelli G, Noble V, Liteplo A, et al. Decreased sensitivity of lung ultrasound limited to the anterior chest in emergency department diagnosis of cardiogenic pulmonary edema: a retrospective analysis. Crit Ultrasound J 2010;2(2):47–52.

16. Ball CG, Kirkpatrick AW, Laupland KB, et al. Factors related to the failure of radiographic recognition of occult posttraumatic pneumothoraces. Am J Surg 2005;189(5):541–6 [discussion: 546].

17. Blaivas M, Lyon M, Duggal S. A prospective comparison of supine chest radiography and bedside ultrasound for the diagnosis of traumatic pneumothorax. Acad Emerg Med 2005;12(9):844–9.

18. Lichtenstein DA, Meziere G, Lascols N, et al. Ultrasound diagnosis of occult pneumothorax. Crit Care Med 2005;33(6):1231–8.

19. Wilkerson RG, Stone MB. Sensitivity of bedside ultrasound and supine anteroposterior chest radiographs for the identification of pneumothorax after blunt trauma. Acad Emerg Med 2010;17(1):11–7.

20. Raja AS, Jacobus CH. How accurate is ultrasonography for excluding pneumothorax? Ann Emerg Med 2013;61(2):207–8.

21. Zhang M, Liu ZH, Yang JX, et al. Rapid detection of pneumothorax by ultrasonography in patients with multiple trauma. Crit Care 2006;10(4):R112.

22. Lyon M, Walton P, Bhalla V, et al. Ultrasound detection of the sliding lung sign by prehospital critical care providers. Am J Emerg Med 2012;30(3):485–8.

23. Kirkpatrick AW, Sirois M, Laupland KB, et al. Hand-held thoracic sonography for detecting post-traumatic pneumothoraces: the Extended Focused Assessment with Sonography for Trauma (EFAST). J Trauma 2004;57(2):288–95.
24. Noble VE. Think ultrasound when evaluating for pneumothorax. J Ultrasound Med 2012;31(3):501–4.
25. Yarmus L, Feller-Kopman D. Pneumothorax in the critically ill patient. Chest 2012;141(4):1098–105.
26. Lichtenstein D, Meziere G, Biderman P, et al. The "lung point": an ultrasound sign specific to pneumothorax. Intensive Care Med 2000;26(10):1434–40.
27. Lichtenstein DA. Ultrasound in the management of thoracic disease. Crit Care Med 2007;35(Suppl 5):S250–61.
28. Slater A, Goodwin M, Anderson KE, et al. COPD can mimic the appearance of pneumothorax on thoracic ultrasound. Chest 2006;129(3):545–50.
29. Blaivas M, Tsung JW. Point-of-care sonographic detection of left endobronchial main stem intubation and obstruction versus endotracheal intubation. J Ultrasound Med 2008;27(5):785–9.
30. Woodring JH. Recognition of pleural effusion on supine radiographs: how much fluid is required? AJR Am J Roentgenol 1984;142(1):59–64.
31. Wong CL, Holroyd-Leduc J, Straus SE. Does this patient have a pleural effusion? JAMA 2009;301(3):309–17.
32. Diaz-Guzman E, Dweik RA. Diagnosis and management of pleural effusions: a practical approach. Compr Ther 2007;33(4):237–46.
33. Rothlin MA, Naf R, Amgwerd M, et al. Ultrasound in blunt abdominal and thoracic trauma. J Trauma 1993;34(4):488–95.
34. Xirouchaki N, Magkanas E, Vaporidi K, et al. Lung ultrasound in critically ill patients: comparison with bedside chest radiography. Intensive Care Med 2011;37(9):1488–93.
35. Zanobetti M, Poggioni C, Pini R. Can chest ultrasonography replace standard chest radiography for evaluation of acute dyspnea in the ED? Chest 2011;139(5):1140–7.
36. Sikora K, Perera P, Mailhot T, et al. Ultrasound for the detection of pleural effusions and guidance of the thoracentesis procedure. ISRN Emergency Medicine 2012. http://dx.doi.org/10.5402/2012/676524.
37. Brooks A, Davies B, Smethhurst M, et al. Emergency ultrasound in the acute assessment of haemothorax. Emerg Med J 2004;21(1):44–6.
38. Atkinson P, Milne J, Loubani O, et al. The V-line: a sonographic aid for the confirmation of pleural fluid. Crit Ultrasound J 2012;4(1):19.
39. Havelock T, Teoh R, Laws D, et al. Pleural procedures and thoracic ultrasound: British Thoracic Society pleural disease guideline 2010. Thorax 2010;65(Suppl 2):i61–76.
40. Lichtenstein D, Hulot JS, Rabiller A, et al. Feasibility and safety of ultrasound-aided thoracentesis in mechanically ventilated patients. Intensive Care Med 1999;25(9):955–8.
41. Jenkins JA, Gharahbaghian L, Doniger SJ, et al. Sonographic Identification of Tube Thoracostomy Study (SITTS): confirmation of intrathoracic placement. West J Emerg Med 2012;13:305–11.
42. Volpicelli G, Elbarbary M, Blaivas M, et al. International evidence-based recommendations for point-of-care lung ultrasound. Intensive Care Med 2012;38(4):577–91.
43. Roger VL, Go AS, Lloyd-Jones DM, et al. Heart disease and stroke statistics–2012 update: a report from the American Heart Association. Circulation 2012;125(1):e2–220.

44. Cardinale L, Volpicelli G, Lamorte A, et al. Revisiting signs, strengths and weaknesses of standard chest radiography in patients of acute dyspnea in the emergency department. J Thorac Dis 2012;4(4):398–407.
45. Green SM, Martinez-Rumayor A, Gregory SA, et al. Clinical uncertainty, diagnostic accuracy, and outcomes in emergency department patients presenting with dyspnea. Arch Intern Med 2008;168(7):741–8.
46. Wang CS, FitzGerald JM, Schulzer M, et al. Does this dyspneic patient in the emergency department have congestive heart failure? JAMA 2005;294(15):1944–56.
47. Soldati G, Copetti R, Sher S. Sonographic interstitial syndrome: the sound of lung water. J Ultrasound Med 2009;28(2):163–74.
48. Agricola E, Bove T, Oppizzi M, et al. "Ultrasound comet-tail figures": a marker of pulmonary edema: a comparative study with wedge pressure and extravascular lung water. Chest 2005;127(5):1690–5.
49. Volpicelli G, Caramello V, Cardinale L, et al. Bedside ultrasound of the lung for the monitoring of acute decompensated heart failure. Am J Emerg Med 2008; 26(5):585–91.
50. Lichtenstein D, Meziere G. A lung ultrasound sign allowing bedside distinction between pulmonary edema and COPD: the comet-tail artifact. Intensive Care Med 1998;24(12):1331–4.
51. Liteplo AS, Marill KA, Villen T, et al. Emergency Thoracic Ultrasound in the Differentiation of the Etiology of Shortness of Breath (ETUDES): sonographic B-lines and N-terminal pro-brain-type natriuretic peptide in diagnosing congestive heart failure. Acad Emerg Med 2009;16(3):201–10.
52. Cardinale L, Volpicelli G, Binello F, et al. Clinical application of lung ultrasound in patients with acute dyspnea: differential diagnosis between cardiogenic and pulmonary causes. Radiol Med 2009;114(7):1053–64.
53. Volpicelli G, Cardinale L, Garofalo G, et al. Usefulness of lung ultrasound in the bedside distinction between pulmonary edema and exacerbation of COPD. Emerg Radiol 2008;15(3):145–51.
54. Wilkins TR, Wilkins RL. Clinical and radiographic evidence of pneumonia. Radiol Technol 2005;77(2):106–10.
55. Blaivas M. Lung ultrasound in evaluation of pneumonia. J Ultrasound Med 2012; 31(6):823–6.
56. Volpicelli G, Caramello V, Cardinale L, et al. Diagnosis of radio-occult pulmonary conditions by real-time chest ultrasonography in patients with pleuritic pain. Ultrasound Med Biol 2008;34(11):1717–23.
57. Lichtenstein DA, Lascols N, Meziere G, et al. Ultrasound diagnosis of alveolar consolidation in the critically ill. Intensive Care Med 2004;30(2):276–81.
58. Reissig A, Copetti R, Mathis G, et al. lung ultrasound in the diagnosis and follow-up of community-acquired pneumonia multicenter study of pneumonia: a prospective, multicenter, diagnostic accuracy study. Chest 2012;142(4):965–72.
59. Lichtenstein D, Mezière G, Seitz J. The dynamic air bronchogram: a lung ultrasound sign of alveolar consolidation ruling out atelectasis. Chest 2009;135(6): 1421–5.
60. Heffner JE, Klein JS, Hampson C. Diagnostic utility and clinical application of imaging for pleural space infections. Chest 2010;137(2):467–79.
61. Werner SL, Smith CE, Goldstein JR, et al. Pilot study to evaluate the accuracy of ultrasonography in confirming endotracheal tube placement. Ann Emerg Med 2007;49(1):75–80.
62. Lichtenstein DA, Lascols N, Prin S, et al. The "lung pulse": an early ultrasound sign of complete atelectasis. Intensive Care Med 2003;29(12):2187–92.

63. Hosseini J, Talebian T. Secondary confirmation of endotracheal tube position by diaphragm motion in right subcostal ultrasound view. IJCIIS 2013;3(2):113–7.
64. Lichtenstein D, Karakitsos D. Integrating lung ultrasound in the hemodynamic evaluation of acute circulatory failure (the fluid administration limited by lung sonography protocol). J Crit Care 2012;27(5):533.e11–9.
65. Khosla R. Bedside Lung Ultrasound in Emergency (BLUE) protocol: a suggestion to modify. Chest 2010;137(6):1487.
66. Manson W, Hafez NM. The rapid assessment of dyspnea with ultrasound: RADIUS. Ultrasound Clin 2011;6(2):261–76.
67. Lichtenstein D. Fluid administration limited by lung sonography: the place of lung ultrasound in assessment of acute circulatory failure (the FALLS-protocol). Expert Rev Respir Med 2012;6(2):155–62.

The FAST and E-FAST in 2013: Trauma Ultrasonography
Overview, Practical Techniques, Controversies, and New Frontiers

Sarah R. Williams, MD*, Phillips Perera, MD, RDMS,
Laleh Gharahbaghian, MD

KEYWORDS

- Trauma • FAST • E-FAST • Ultrasound • Point-of-care • Hemoperitoneum
- Hemothorax • Pneumothorax

KEY POINTS

- The FAST (Focused Assessment with Sonography in Trauma) and E-FAST (Extended Focused Assessment with Sonography in Trauma) examinations provide critical information during the real-time evaluation of complex trauma patients, directly at the bedside.
- The FAST examination can identify free fluid suggestive of abdominal solid-organ injury, hemothorax, or pericardial fluid collections.
- The sensitivity of E-FAST for pneumothorax and hemothorax is superior to that of chest radiography.
- To use the FAST and E-FAST optimally, physicians must be familiar with both their strengths and their weaknesses.

INTRODUCTION: TRAUMA "EPIDEMIC"

Trauma continues to be a major cause of morbidity and mortality worldwide. The percentage of global deaths attributable to injuries in 2010 (5.1 million deaths) was higher than 2 decades earlier. This trend was driven primarily by a worldwide 46% increase in deaths caused by motor vehicle collisions and from falls.[1]

In the United States, vigorous safety regulations as well as an interdisciplinary trauma care systems have provided relative protection from fatalities, which were at a 60-year low in 2011. However, early statistics from 2012 suggest that numbers are again on the rise (an increase of 7.1%).[2] Among the young (aged 0–19 years),

Division of Emergency Medicine, Department of Surgery, Stanford University Medical Center, 300 Pasteur Drive Alway Building, M121, Stanford, CA 93405, USA
* Corresponding author.
E-mail address: srwilliams@stanford.edu

Crit Care Clin 30 (2014) 119–150
http://dx.doi.org/10.1016/j.ccc.2013.08.005
0749-0704/14/$ – see front matter © 2014 Elsevier Inc. All rights reserved.
criticalcare.theclinics.com

unintentional injuries continue to be the leading cause of death, with approximately 12,000 annual fatalities. However, more than 9 million young persons present to emergency departments (EDs) yearly with nonfatal injuries.[3] Unfortunately, violent injuries also continue to be a major cause of death and morbidity; an estimated 50,000 persons die yearly in the United States from these injuries.[4]

Overall, unintentional and violence-related injuries together caused 48.5% of the deaths of persons aged 1 to 44 years of age in the United States: more fatalities than by infectious disease and noncommunicable diseases combined.[5]

With American EDs already beyond capacity[6] and trauma rates increasing worldwide, these statistics emphasize the continued importance of optimizing trauma care with resource-efficient and cost-efficient modalities. There is also now significant concern over radiation levels involved in standard imaging modalities such as computed tomography (CT). The FAST (Focused Assessment with Sonography in Trauma) examination addresses many of these issues in the evaluation of chest and abdominal trauma.

FAST: INTRODUCTION AND ENDORSEMENT

Over the last 2 decades the FAST examination, and thereafter the E-FAST (Extended Focused Assessment with Sonography in Trauma) examination, have transformed the management of trauma patients in the United States. In 2013 and beyond, it is critical for clinicians to be adept at its use, while also understanding its limitations. The American College of Emergency Physicians (ACEP) recognized its critical importance in the landmark 2008 ACEP Ultrasound Guidelines.[7] These guidelines were also recognized in 2011 by the American Institute of Ultrasound in Medicine (AIUM).[8] The American College of Surgeons has adopted the FAST into the Advanced Trauma Life Support (ATLS) protocol. The ninth edition of ATLS has DPL (diagnostic peritoneal lavage) as only an optional skill station, owing to the widespread utilization of the FAST examination.[9] This situation is remarkable when one considers that before 1995, abdominal trauma was being evaluated with the invasive diagnostic peritoneal lavage (DPL) test[10] at most trauma centers. Following several seminal studies, this approach to trauma patients radically changed. Trauma ultrasonography is one of the key applications of point-of-care ultrasound.[11]

Cases

Three cases are presented, each highlighting important aspects of the E-FAST examination. These cases are referred to throughout the article.

Case 1

History and physical examination. A 9-year-old boy who was involved in a serious rollover minivan crash presents via paramedic transport to your Emergency Department (ED). There were fatalities on scene. The child has an altered mental status and is unable to actively participate in the examination. The vital signs include: blood pressure (BP) 88/60 mm Hg, heart rate (HR) 122 beats per minute, respiratory rate (RR) 25 breaths per minute, pulse oxygenation (POX) 99% on supplemental oxygen. The primary survey is significant for a patent airway, ashen skin appearance with poor capillary refill and a right leg below-the-knee amputation with ongoing hemorrhage despite a tourniquet. The Glasgow Coma Scale (GCS) is 14, due to the presence of confusion. Chest and abdominal examinations are significant for mild diffuse tenderness to palpation.

ED course/imaging. Crystalloid and blood were administered. It was unclear if the patient's shock state was due to the hemorrhage from the leg amputation or from another potential source. Bedside E-FAST was immediately performed and was positive for free fluid in the abdomen and pelvis. Due to the patient's unstable hemodynamic status, CT scan was deferred and the patient was taken immediately to the operating room for abdominal laparotomy, as well as for definitive control of the hemorrhage from the amputation.

Case 2

History and physical examination. A 23-year-old male bicyclist arrives to your ED via paramedic transport after being thrown while traveling at a high rate of speed down a hill. He was wearing a helmet. On primary survey, he is alert and awake, appropriately interactive with GCS 15, and in no acute respiratory distress. His vital signs include BP 95/50 mm Hg, HR 110 beats per minute, RR 20 breaths per minute, POX 98% on room air. On further examination, he has diffuse abdominal tenderness to palpation without rebound or guarding. The pelvis is tender diffusely. The remainder of the examination is within normal limits.

ED course/imaging. Resuscitation was initiated with intravenous fluids. Chest radiograph (CXR) and pelvis X-ray were ordered. Bedside E-FAST was negative for free fluid within the thorax, abdomen and pelvis. No pneumothorax was noted in either the right or left thoracic cavities. Repeat vital signs were taken: BP 75/52 mm Hg, HR 120 beats per minute. Pelvis radiograph demonstrated an open book pelvic fracture. A pelvic binder was immediately placed and massive transfusion protocol was initiated. A repeat E-FAST was negative. After discussion with both orthopedics and interventional radiology (IR), the patient was taken to the IR suite, where hemostasis was achieved after pelvic vessel embolization.

Case 3

History and physical examination. A 55-year-old male was transported by paramedics following a motor vehicle crash. The paramedics reported that the vehicle had a moderate amount of damage. On their examination, the patient had decreased breath sounds on the right side of the chest. He also appeared intoxicated. On ED trauma survey, the vital signs included: BP 150/92 mm Hg, HR 95 beats per minute, RR 14 breaths per minute and POX 92% on room air. The patient was intoxicated, but following commands. He had a patent airway. Breath sounds were decreased at both lung bases. The chest and abdomen were non-tender to palpation.

ED course/imaging. A CXR was ordered. The trauma surgery team initially wanted to place a chest tube on the patient's right side, given the history of decreased breath sounds and relative hypoxia. However, E-FAST was immediately performed and demonstrated positive lung sliding and the presence of comet-tail artifacts on examination of both the right and left thoracic cavities. The chest tube was deferred. Supplemental oxygen was administered, with improvement of the POX to 100%. Subsequent imaging with CXR, followed by CT scan of the chest, demonstrated no pneumothorax. The patient was observed, made a complete recovery, and was discharged from the ED.

Utility of the FAST Examination: Evidence

As these cases demonstrate, the management of trauma patients is highly complex. Patients often arrive with multiple injuries and/or are in shock. Patients may have altered mental status resulting from head injury, intoxication, or cerebral hypoperfusion; they often have distracting injuries, which further confounds the ability to diagnose their injury pattern with physical examination alone. Several studies have shown the physical examination to be highly inaccurate in trauma patients.[12–14]

The FAST examination is a noninvasive test that can be done rapidly at the bedside to address a specific clinical question. The examination evaluates for the presence of intra-peritoneal free fluid in the abdomen and pelvis. In addition, the cardiac views allow for detection of cardiac injury and pericardial effusion. The E-FAST allows for the assessment of a hemothorax or pneumothorax, and has become an accepted standard of care in the resuscitation of the injured patient.[15] The FAST exam has been shown to have good to outstanding sensitivity in many studies (73%–99%).[16–21] A recent study of more than 4000 patients with blunt trauma by Lee and colleagues[22] had a sensitivity of 85%, regardless of blood pressure. In this series the specificity was 96% and overall accuracy 95%. A recent meta-analysis of 62 trials (including more than 18,000 patients) using FAST showed a pooled sensitivity of 78.9% and specificity of 99.2%, demonstrating that while the FAST exam may miss smaller amounts of fluid in some trauma patients, a positive exam is highly accurate for significant intra-peritoneal injury and can be reliably used in clinical practice.[23]

Quinn and Sinert[24] recently performed a systematic review of the literature on penetrating torso injury. These investigators found that a positive study had a high incidence of intra-abdominal injury, and recommended exploratory laparotomy in these patients. However, a negative study cannot be used as a single rule-out tool.

The FAST examination is particularly powerful in patients with precordial penetrating wounds and in hypotensive patients with blunt torso trauma, with sensitivity of 100%.[25] In this subset of patients, immediate surgical intervention is indicated in patients with a positive FAST.[25–29]

It is extremely important to remember that the abdominal components of the FAST are specifically designed to evaluate for free fluid suggestive of hemoperitoneum, a condition most commonly resulting from injuries to the spleen or liver, among other pathology. The FAST exam is not designed to reliably detect injuries to the solid organs, intestine, mesentery, diaphragm, nor the retroperitoneal hemorrhage that may occur with pelvic fractures (as in Case 2). Further details are given in the Pitfalls section. Some studies suggest the utility of contrast agents that can improve visualization of solid-organ injury, and this is discussed in the section New Frontiers.

Feasibility

Several studies support both the feasibility and the rapid nature of performing the FAST examination. The entire scan can be performed in around 3 to 4 minutes.[30–33] Additional benefits include the lack of ionizing radiation and the ability to easily repeat the examination, especially in cases of high clinical suspicion or a change in clinical status. This aspect is particularly important, considering that approximately one-third of stable patients with significant intra-abdominal injury may not have significant free fluid evident on initial evaluation.[34] Potentially unstable patients can also be assessed in the ED or other critical care areas, decreasing the risk of transport.

The number of proctored examinations required for competence has been a matter of debate, as numbers established previously by imaging organizations did not take into account several aspects of the FAST: (1) the rapid point-of-care nature of the study, (2) the single "yes/no" binary quality of the study outcome, and (3) the fact that clinical correlation was being immediately applied. Shackford and colleagues[35] found an initial error rate of 17% in nonradiologist clinical sonographers, which decreased to 5% after 10 examinations. Jang and colleagues[36] found that the incidence of technical errors of emergency physicians learning to perform FAST improved with hands-on experience. Noninterpretable or misinterpreted views occurred in 24% of examinations for those performing their first 10 examinations, 3.6% for those performing their 41st to 50th examinations, and 0% for those performing their 71st to 75th examinations. Interpretive skills improved more rapidly than image acquisition skills. The ACEP Guidelines recommend at least 25 to 50 studies in this core US application.[7]

PITFALLS OF FAST
Quantity of Fluid

The FAST examination is designed to evaluate for intraperitoneal free fluid. Volumes of less than 400 mL in the right upper quadrant (RUQ) have been hard to distinguish. In a study on infused volumes of DPL fluid, Branney and colleagues[37] found that only 10% of participants performing FAST could detect fluid volumes of less than 400 mL. The mean volume detected was 619 mL. This volume fits in well with the classes of hemorrhage described in ATLS, corresponding to a Class 3 hemorrhage (loss of 30%–40% of blood volume) and potential hypotension.[9] After all, this is where the FAST has shown the greatest benefit in trauma care. The pelvic views of the FAST have shown better sensitivity, although they are limited if the bladder is empty or if a Foley catheter has already been placed. Von Kuenssberg, Jehle and colleagues[38] found that the mean minimal volume of fluid needed for pelvic ultrasonography detection by the examiner was 157 mL.

Therefore, the FAST examination cannot be used as a diagnostic test to rule out small amounts of intra-peritoneal hemorrhage in all trauma patients. However, as discussed above, its utility chiefly lies in the ability to rapidly detect the significant amount of blood that can result in hemodynamic instability in the trauma patient. Given the relative benefits of the FAST exam, DPL has been relegated to a very rare procedure, especially since this test is over-sensitive and has resulted in unnecessary surgeries in the past. CT remains the gold standard for the detection of intra-abdominal injury and free fluid, although the discriminatory zone for this test is estimated to be 100–250 cc of fluid and CT may also potentially miss some smaller quantities of bleeding.[39] Furthermore, CT may miss clinically significant injuries that may result in little free abdominal bleeding, such as mesenteric, intestinal and pancreatic injuries.[40]

Solid-Organ Injury

Ultrasonography cannot reliably grade solid-organ injuries that do not result in significant hemoperitoneum.[41–44] CT imaging and/or careful serial abdominal examinations remain indicated to further delineate these injuries in high-risk patients. See also section on Pitfalls and Negative FAST: Clinical Judgment and Serial Examinations Remain Paramount, below.

Delayed Presentation

Free fluid only remains echolucent, or anechoic (black), on ultrasound until it begins to clot. It can then become more echogenic (bright) and more difficult to differentiate from the surrounding tissue. Therefore, extra care must be taken in assessing patients with a delayed presentation after trauma, as the FAST may be falsely reassuring.

Pelvic Fracture/Pelvic Trauma

In cases where pelvic fracture is suspected, ultrasonography cannot reliably evaluate for hemorrhage from a pelvic-fracture source, as in Case 2 (see also **Table 1** for further details). A rapid pelvic radiograph is critical in this patient population. Also, if free fluid is present the FAST cannot delineate between free fluid from a bladder rupture and hemoperitoneum. Further imaging is warranted in this patient subset.[45,46]

As many trauma patients have hemorrhage from multiple sources, many trauma teams use the FAST to evaluate for evidence of intra-abdominal free fluid even with pelvic fracture, as the optimal approach in these patients will be both interventional radiology (to embolize the pelvic vessels) and concurrent laparotomy.

Table 1
Summary of studies using FAST and their key findings

Authors,[Ref.] Year	Study Design and Findings	Key Points
Branney et al,[54] 1997	Prospective analysis of blunt abdominal trauma patients. 486 patients were enrolled in KCP including FAST. This group was compared with historical cohort. DPL was reduced from 17% to 4%; CT was reduced from 56% to 26%. US examinations were used exclusively in 65% of the patients	A US-based KCP resulted in significant reductions in the use of invasive DPL and costly CT scanning without risk to the patient
Blackbourne et al,[34] 2004	Prospective observational study of 547 trauma patients with both initial and secondary US within 24 h of admission. The accuracy of initial US was 92.1% and 96.7% on the secondary US. No clinically significant hemoperitoneum developed in any patients with negative secondary US after 4 h	A second FAST examination significantly improves accuracy. Consider repeat US after an observation period of 4 h
Sarkisian et al,[55] 1991	US was performed as the primary screening procedure in 400 of 750 mass casualty patients with trauma in the first 72 h after the 1988 Armenian earthquake. Average time per patient was 4 min. More than 130 follow-up US were also performed. 12.8% of patients had trauma-associated pathology, with a 1% false-negative rate	The first article showing the utility of trauma US in mass casualty settings where resource utilization is paramount
Plummer et al,[26] 1992	A 10-year retrospective review of outcomes of patients with penetrating cardiac injuries. 49 patients were reviewed. 28 of these received immediate bedside echo; 21 did not. The probability of survival in each group was 34.2% and 31.8%, respectively. The actual survival was 100% in the echo group and 57.1% in the nonecho group. Neurologic outcome was also better in the echo group	An early important study showing significantly enhanced survival in patients with penetrating cardiac injury who received early echo
Ma et al,[32] 1995	Data from a prior prospective US study of 245 trauma patients with blunt or penetrating trauma injuries was retrospectively analyzed to determine if a multiple-view FAST examination had higher sensitivity than a single view. The multiple-view technique had a sensitivity of 87%. The Morison view alone had a sensitivity of only 51%. Gold standards were exploratory laparotomy, CT, or DPL	This early study on FAST showed the need for a multiple views to achieve acceptable sensitivity

Friese et al,[46] 2007	Retrospective review of 146 patients with pelvic fracture with at least 1 of the following risk factors for hemorrhage: age ≥55, evidence of hemorrhagic shock (SBP <100), or unstable fracture pattern. 126 of these patients had a FAST examination performed; 104 had confirmatory CT or exploratory laparotomy. Sensitivity and specificity of US were 26% and 96%, respectively	A negative FAST examination does not preclude the need for laparotomy or pelvic angiography in patients with pelvic fracture at risk for hemorrhage
Rozycki et al,[25] 1998	FAST examinations were performed on 1540 patients with precordial or transthoracic wounds or blunt abdominal trauma. Patients with positive US for hemopericardium underwent immediate surgery; patients with positive US for hemoperitoneum received either a CT (if stable) or immediate celiotomy if unstable. There were 1440 true-negative results, 80 true-positive results, 16 false negatives, and 4 false positives. Overall sensitivity was 83.3% and specificity was 99.7%. US had 100% sensitivity for patients with precordial or transthoracic wounds and hypotensive patients with blunt abdominal trauma	Recommended that US should be the initial diagnostic test for evaluating patients with precordial wounds and blunt truncal injuries. Also recommended immediate surgical intervention in patients with positive US with precordial wounds or blunt torso trauma patients with hypotension
Nishijima et al,[56] 2012	Extensive meta-analysis of literature since 1950 on intra-abdominal injuries; included 12 studies on clinical findings and 22 studies on bedside US. The presence of intraperitoneal fluid or organ injury on bedside US was more accurate than any history or physical examination findings (LR 30). These findings included US, seat-belt sign, hypotension, abdominal distension, and guarding. Importantly, the absence of abdominal tenderness did not rule out an intra-abdominal injury	Important meta-analysis confirming high accuracy of US in trauma. However, a negative result does not rule out injury; the ideal combination of variables needs further study

Abbreviations: CT, computed tomography; DPL, diagnostic peritoneal lavage; KCP, key clinical pathway; LR, likelihood ratio; SBP, systolic blood pressure; US, ultrasonography.

Retroperitoneal Hemorrhage

Retroperitoneal hemorrhage is poorly visualized on ultrasonography.[43,47] Retroperitoneal bleeding can result from a multitude of sources: pelvic fracture, injury to the great vessels (inferior vena cava [IVC] and aorta), and renal injuries. If the hemorrhage remains encapsulated in the retroperitoneal space and does not flow into the abdominal/pelvic compartments, the FAST can remain negative.

Positive FAST That May Not Be Due To Hemoperitoneum

In unstable patients with positive FAST examinations in whom there is a diagnostic dilemma regarding the type of free fluid present (ie, patients with a history of ascites or a concern about bladder rupture), an emergency bedside paracentesis may be performed under ultrasound guidance.[33] In these cases, the color of the aspirate will be immediately useful (red for blood, yellow for urine or ascites).

Negative FAST in an Unstable Patient

In patients with hemodynamic instability for whom the FAST examination is negative and the patient is too unstable to go to CT, a diagnostic peritoneal aspirate (DPA) may be useful if the cause of shock remains unknown. This technique is a modified version of the DPL, which has now been largely replaced by the FAST examination. In this procedure, the abdomen is aspirated for the presence of gross blood. No lavage is done. If positive, the patient should go immediately to the operating room.[48]

False-Positive FAST

Occasionally, false-positive FAST examinations occur, which can result from misinterpreting fluid-filled bowel as free fluid.[49] If in doubt, watch for peristalsis, and/or repeat the examination to ensure the fluid pocket(s) are in the appropriate tissue planes. If the gallbladder or renal cysts are prominent in the Morison's pouch, these can also be interpreted as a positive FAST. The key is the contained and circular appearance of cysts and body structures as opposed to the free-flowing appearance of blood. The fat surrounding the kidney in some obese patients may also occasionally be misinterpreted as free fluid.[50] Evaluating for the double line sign around the kidneys may be helpful in differentiating some cases of prominent perinephric fat, where this finding is noted, from free abdominal fluid.[50]

False-Negative FAST

False negative FAST examinations may occur when the scan is performed soon after the injury and the volume of free fluid is small. Repeating the exam at regular intervals, or especially if the clinical status changes, is an excellent approach to increasing the sensitivity of the exam and avoiding a false negative result.[34] Many times an initial negative exam may convert to a positive one as further fluid accumulates during resuscitation with intravenous fluids and/or blood. Delayed presentation of injury can also allow time for blood to clot, changing the echogenicity of blood and decreasing its tendency to layer out; additional care needs to be taken in this patient subset.

Laselle and colleagues[51] provide an excellent overview of false-negative FAST scans. These investigators studied 332 patients with a median injury severity score of 27. Of these, 49% had a false-negative FAST. Patients with severe head injuries and minor abdominal injuries were more likely to have a false-negative than a true-positive FAST. However, they also found that patients with liver, spleen, or abdominal vascular injuries are less likely to have false-negative FAST scans. Of importance, adverse outcomes were not associated with false-negative FASTs. In fact, patients with false-negative FAST scans were less likely to have a therapeutic laparotomy.

Negative FAST: Clinical Judgment and Serial Examinations Remain Paramount

In patients with a significant mechanism or concern, clinical judgment must prevail; reaching "premature closure" with a negative FAST examination can result in significant morbidity and mortality. In one study, 60% of deaths resulted largely from delayed treatment of splenic or other abdominal injuries.[52] By comparison, a large study of almost 4000 patients showed that a combination of careful negative serial examinations and negative screening ultrasonograms, over an observation period of at least 12 to 24 hours, virtually excluded abdominal injury.[53]

Summary Table: FAST Studies

A summary of some of the key original FAST studies, including study design, patient population, and key findings, are presented in **Table 1**. An important recent meta-analysis is also included.

TUTORIAL: FAST

When performing a FAST examination, it is important to remember that free fluid will first collect in the most dependent regions of the abdomen and pelvis. In the supine patient, the most dependent portion of the abdominal cavity is the right upper quadrant area region around Morison's pouch.[57] In the pelvis, the retro-vesicular space in the male and the pelvic cul-de-sac in the female are the most dependent regions. Unfortunately, one single view is not sufficient to rule out free fluid.[52]

If the trauma patient has been in an upright position, the free fluid may be more evident within the pelvis. It is critical to perform the exam of the pelvis prior to placing a Foley catheter, as a full bladder serves as the acoustic window for the imaging of free fluid in this area. Another potential pitfall is that rolling the patient to inspect the back prior to the FAST exam may disturb the normal flow of blood and limit the sensitivity of the exam. Positioning the patient in Trendelenburg may improve the sensitivity of the right upper quadrant FAST views by up to one third, through the shifting of blood from the pelvis into the right upper quadrant.[58]

Performing the FAST Examination: Technique

Evaluate all 4 regions (RUQ, left upper quadrant [LUQ], cardiac, and suprapubic views) with a low-frequency (3–5 MHz) probe; this can be a small footprint phased-array (which aids in evaluating between the ribs) or a curved probe (**Fig. 1**). The convention is to orient the probe marker to the patient's right (for transverse views) or head (for longitudinal or coronal views). The ultrasound machine should be set to abdominal presets.

Intraperitoneal fluid is anechoic (black); it appears as a black stripe on standard machine settings. Intraparenchymal or clotted blood can become more echogenic and heterogeneous. This caveat is important, and should be considered if presentation is delayed and no gross free fluid is evident.

If suspicion for hemorrhage is high, the patient should be placed in Trendelenburg.[58] Increased fluid collection with ongoing hemorrhage will increase the likelihood of visualization (especially after resuscitation with crystalloid and blood products). In high-risk patients, a CT scan should be strongly considered if the patient is stable.

Cardiac view

For the cardiac view (Please refer to Cardiac Echocardiography article by Perera and colleagues elsewhere in this issue), indications include assessment for free fluid within

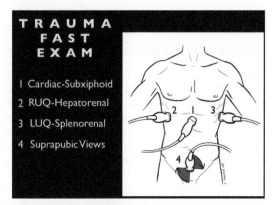

Fig. 1. Probe placement for FAST examination. In penetrating trauma, position 1 (cardiac) should be performed first, to rule out pericardial tamponade. In blunt trauma, position 2 (right upper quadrant [RUQ]) should be performed first, as this is usually the most sensitive view for hemoperitoneum. LUQ, left upper quadrant.

the pericardium to evaluate for tamponade. It can also be used to evaluate for cardiac activity in cases of traumatic cardiac arrest.

- Technique
  a. Place the probe just inferior to the xiphoid process with the indicator toward the right and angle it up toward the left shoulder.
  b. Ensure visualization of the entire heart, including the posterior pericardium, as pericardial effusions start here; this can be done by increasing the depth on the ultrasound system or having the patient breathe in deeply (**Fig. 2**).
  c. If you are unable to use this view because of habitus or pain, use the parasternal long-axis view. Place the probe between the second and fourth intercostal spaces on the anterior chest wall just to the left of the sternum, with the indicator toward the patient's left hip (see also the articles on echo and resuscitation elsewhere in this issue) (**Figs. 3–5**).

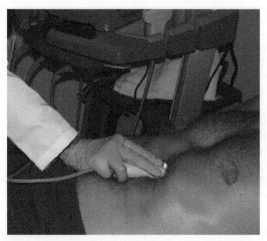

Fig. 2. Probe placement: subxiphoid (subcostal) view.

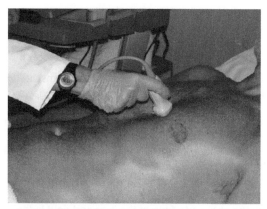

Fig. 3. Probe placement: parasternal long-axis view.

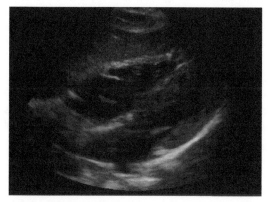

Fig. 4. Negative subxiphoid cardiac view.

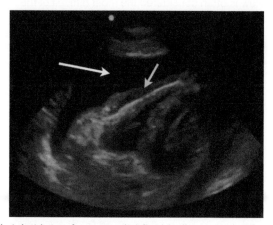

Fig. 5. Positive subxiphoid view for pericardial fluid (*yellow arrow*). Of note, a clot sealing a penetrating wound in the right ventricle is also present (*blue arrow*).

Right upper quadrant (including Morison's pouch)

This view assesses the potential space between the liver and kidney in the RUQ, using the liver as the sonographic window. It also assesses the regions just above and below the diaphragm and the upper portion of the paracolic gutter on the right.

- Indications: assessment for hemoperitoneum and hemothorax.
- This view is the most sensitive of the abdominal FAST views for free intraperitoneal fluid.
- However, it is imperative to complete the FAST if this view is negative.
- Technique
  a. Place the probe in the right anterior to midaxillary line between the seventh and eighth interspaces (**Figs. 6** and **7**).
  b. It is important to visualize the diaphragm to assess for free fluid in the thorax (position 1 in **Fig. 6**).
  c. Fan through the entire interface of the liver and right kidney through at least 2 respiratory cycles (position 2 in **Fig. 6**).
  d. Assess the caudal tip of the liver, as small fluid collections start here; this is depicted by position 3 in **Fig. 6**. Effectively this is the beginning of the right paracolic gutter, and fluid will often pool here before entering the Morison's pouch. Historically, the right and left paracolic views were part of some FAST protocols. However, this caudal view of the tip of the liver is the most sensitive of these views and maximizes the entire RUQ view (**Figs. 8–10**).

Left upper quadrant

This view assesses the potential space between the spleen and the kidney in the LUQ, using the spleen as the sonographic window. It also assesses the regions just above and below the diaphragm and the upper portion of the paracolic gutter on the left.

- Indications: assessment for hemoperitoneum and hemothorax.
- Technique
  a. Place the probe in the left posterior-axillary line between the seventh and eighth interspaces (**Figs. 11** and **12**).
  b. Fan through the entire interface of the spleen and the left kidney.
  c. The spleen is a smaller sonographic window than the liver. Usually the probe needs to be placed both more cephalad and more posterior to obtain a good view. This view is often considered the most difficult of the FAST views, owing to the smaller size of the spleen (in reference to the liver). In addition, air and

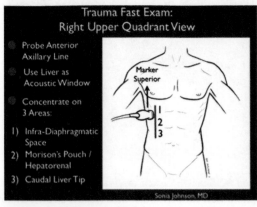

Fig. 6. Placement of probe for RUQ evaluation.

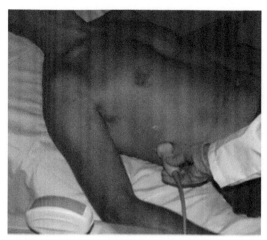

Fig. 7. Probe placement: RUQ view.

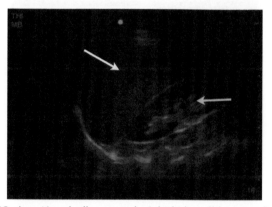

Fig. 8. Normal RUQ view. Liver (*yellow arrow*); right kidney (*blue arrow*).

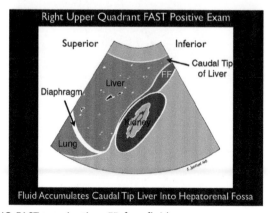

Fig. 9. Positive RUQ FAST examination. FF, free fluid.

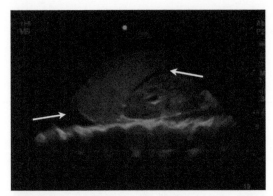

Fig. 10. Abnormal RUQ view: free fluid (*arrows*) in Morison's pouch (between liver and kidney) and in the chest cephalad to the diaphragm (hemothorax).

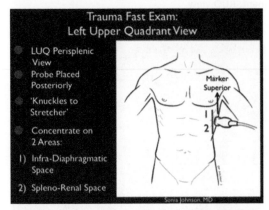

Fig. 11. Placement of probe for left upper quadrant (LUQ) evaluation.

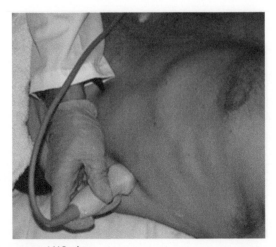

Fig. 12. Probe placement: LUQ view.

gas in the stomach and colon can obstruct this view. Positioning the probe in a more superior and posterior position (relative to the right), with the examiner's knuckles touching the gurney, can often facilitate improved views by moving the probe around the intestinal gas and fluid. In addition, turning the probe into a more oblique orientation parallel to the ribs (with the indicator dot oriented superiorly and posteriorly) can allow for better imaging by avoiding interference from the rib shadows. Aiming the probe posteriorly also minimizes interference from the stomach.

d. Fluid flows differently in the LUQ than in the RUQ. The phrenicolic ligament limits the flow of free fluid down the left paracolic gutter. It is extremely important to visualize the interface between the diaphragm and the spleen to avoid false negatives. It is helpful to use respirations to visualize the subdiaphragmatic space.

e. Visualize the space above the diaphragm to check for free fluid in the thorax.

f. Complete the left upper quadrant exam by moving the probe more inferiorly to assess the inferior pole of the kidney and the area between the spleen and the kidney (**Figs. 13–15**).

Suprapubic (pelvic) view

This view assesses the pelvis for free fluid, using the bladder as the sonographic window.

- Indications: assessment for free fluid in pelvis. Note that this view cannot be used to rule out hemorrhage from a pelvic fracture source (see Pitfalls).
- A small amount of free fluid in women can be physiologic; clinical correlation is important.
- Technique
  a. Place the probe just above the pubic symphysis and aim down toward the feet, fanning through the bladder in both longitudinal and transverse orientations (**Figs. 16–18**).
  b. In the female, free pelvic fluid will first be seen in the cul-de-sac, posterior to the uterus. Larger amounts of fluid will collect behind the bladder, both anteriorly and posteriorly to the uterus. In the male, free pelvic fluid will be seen in the retrovesical space (**Figs. 19** and **20**).

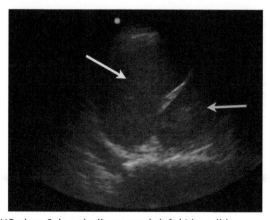

Fig. 13. Normal LUQ view. Spleen (*yellow arrow*); left kidney (*blue arrow*).

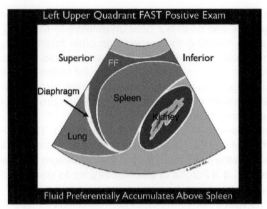

Fig. 14. Positive LUQ FAST examination. FF, free fluid.

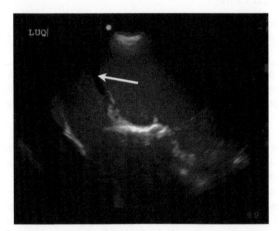

Fig. 15. Abnormal LUQ view: free fluid (*arrow*) in spleen in a pediatric trauma patient (e.g., Case 1).

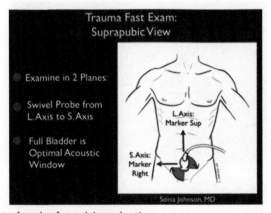

Fig. 16. Placement of probe for pelvis evaluation.

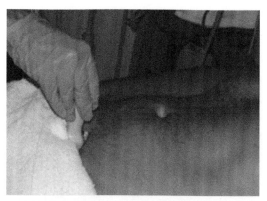

Fig. 17. Probe placement: suprapubic.

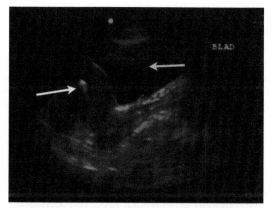

Fig. 18. Negative suprapubic FAST view (female): no significant free fluid. Note that an intrauterine device is present (*yellow arrow*). Bladder (*blue arrow*).

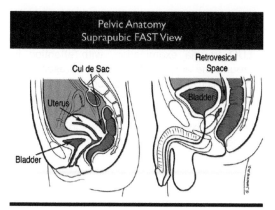

Fig. 19. Pelvic anatomy for suprapubic FAST examination.

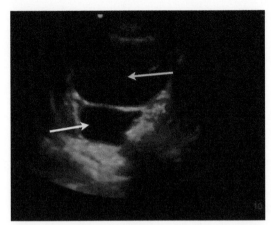

Fig. 20. Positive suprapubic view: free fluid (*yellow arrow*) behind the bladder (*blue arrow*).

c. The term "double-wall sign" is often used to describe a positive pelvic FAST in a male. Free fluid outside the bladder will illuminate the outer bladder wall, and urine will illuminate the inner bladder wall (see **Fig. 20**).

d. Pitfalls for a false-positive pelvic scan include ovarian cysts in women, seminal vesicles in men, an enlarged rectum, or prominent prostate.

e. Filling the bladder (either with hydration or retrograde fluid infiltration through a Foley catheter) can improve visualization, although this technique has generally fallen out of practice.

E-FAST
Background

For the purposes of this article, this section discusses the evaluation of the chest for hemothorax and pneumothorax on extended FAST (E-FAST). The key is to consider using ultrasonography of the chest for the evaluation of pneumothorax and clinically significant hemothorax as part of the FAST examination. For further discussion of thoracic ultrasound, please refer to the article by Lobo and colleagues elsewhere in this issue.

Hemothorax

The evaluation for hemothorax is performed by using the same windows and probe as for the RUQ and LUQ trauma examination, with attention focused on above the diaphragm and around the adjacent lung. Lung ultrasonography appears to be as sensitive as or more sensitive than chest radiography (CXR) for the evaluation of hemothorax.[20,21] In a recent prospective study by Zanobetti and colleagues[59] on a group of nontrauma patients with symptomatic dyspnea from a pleural effusion, there was a high concordance between ultrasonography and radiography for pleural effusion. However, when there was disagreement, ultrasonography was more accurate than CXR in distinguishing pleural effusion, and much faster to obtain.

Pneumothorax

The evaluation for pneumothorax is optimally performed with a high-frequency linear probe. The probe is positioned in the second intercostal space in the mid-clavicular line with the indicator marker oriented toward the patient's head. The exam utilizes both gray-scale B-mode imaging and M-mode imaging to best demonstrate lung sliding. Case 3 illustrates an example of a chest tube that was avoided in a trauma patient by using rapid bedside ultrasonography.

E-FAST for pneumothorax shows great benefit, as the incidence of occult pneumothoraces approaches 15% among injured patients undergoing CT. Remarkably, up to 76% of all pneumothoraces (detected by CT) may be occult on supine CXR with real-time interpretation by trauma teams.[60] The E-FAST has a greater sensitivity than supine CXR for pneumothorax,[61,62] and may decrease the need to perform chest CT.[63] It has also been shown to be superior to upright CXR in a series of postbiopsy patients with iatrogenic pneumothorax.[64] Chest ultrasonography as part of the E-FAST detects up to 92% to 100% of all pneumothoraces.[60]

PITFALLS OF E-FAST
Choice of Gold-Standard Effects Sensitivity

Ultrasound has been shown to have a sensitivity that equals or exceeds that of CXR for detection of hemothorax. CT imaging remains the gold standard against which all other imaging modalities for pleural fluid are compared. However, ultrasound has been found to have a discriminatory threshold that differs only by 10–50 ml when compared to CT imaging. One study stated that ultrasound had a poor sensitivity for the evaluation of clinically insignificant small hemothoraces as compared to CT imaging.[65] However, due to the ability of ultrasound to detect as little as 20–50 ml of fluid, one may question the study premise of comparing the 2 imaging modalities in their ability to detect pleural fluid that was not deemed clinically significant.

Loculated Pneumothorax and Subcutaneous Emphysema

Loculated traumatic pneumothoraces that are not near the second intercostal space may be difficult to identify using standard E-FAST views.[64] If there is high suspicion for pneumothorax and the E-FAST is negative, the probe should be used to evaluate additional areas of the chest in a manner similar to evaluation for the lung point.[63] Subcutaneous emphysema can interfere with the visualization of the pleural line; however, in these cases pneumothorax is clinically extremely likely.[66]

False Positives for Pneumothorax

False positives in the evaluation of pneumothorax can be caused by the presence of bullae, adhesions, and contusions.[67] Therefore, particular care should be taken in patients with a history of chronic obstructive pulmonary disease or previous lung abnormality.

Summary Table: E-FAST: Hemothorax and Pneumothorax Studies

A summary of some of the key E-FAST studies, including study design, patient population, and key findings, is presented in **Table 2**. An important recent meta-analysis is also included.

TUTORIAL: E-FAST

- Indications: blunt or penetrating trauma to chest with concern for hemothorax or pneumothorax.

Table 2
Summary of E-FAST hemothorax and pneumothorax studies and their key findings

Authors,[Ref.] Year	Study Design and Findings	Key Points
Blaivas et al,[61] 2005	Prospective study of 176 trauma patients receiving CT imaging including lung windows. Attending emergency physicians performed bedside trauma US to determine the presence of lung sliding. Portable supine AP CXRs were reviewed by attending trauma surgeons, blinded to the results of the US. CT or air release on chest-tube placement were considered gold standards. US was 98.1% sensitive and 99.2% specific for PTX. Conversely, CXR had only 75.5% sensitivity, with specificity of 100%. US also allowed for differentiation between small, medium, and large PTX	CXR may miss small to moderate PTX in trauma patients, especially if the PTX is anterior. This study shows that US as part of the E-FAST is more sensitive than supine CXR for identifying traumatic PTX
Ma & Mateer,[20] 1997	Retrospective analysis of a prior prospective study of trauma US on 245 adult patients with blunt and penetrating torso trauma to determine utility of US in assessing hemothorax. The trauma US included evaluation for pleural fluid; US interpretations were recorded before other test results were available. These were compared with CXR and CT interpreted by radiologists (who were not blinded to patient outcome). 5 patients were excluded because of chest-tube placement before the US was done. 26 of 240 study patients had hemothorax confirmed by tube thoracostomy or CT. Both US and CXR showed equivalent sensitivities and specificities for hemothorax, at 96.2% and 100%, respectively	Suggests that US is at least as sensitive and specific as CXR in identification of hemothorax. It may expedite this diagnosis in major trauma patients
Abboud & Kendall,[65] 2003	Prospective study of blunt-trauma patients who underwent CT of the chest, abdomen, or both. Before CT, US was performed to evaluate for free fluid in the thorax. The ED US was 12.5% sensitive and 98.4% specific when using CT as the gold standard. US was limited in its ability to pick up small-volume hemothorax. Of note, patients who had small effusions on CT did not have clinically relevant consequences	US is at least as good as CXR for hemothorax (as above), but not as sensitive as CT for small-volume hemothorax of unclear clinical significance

Lichtenstein et al,[63] 2005	Retrospective study of 200 consecutive undifferentiated ICU patients who received a chest CT in addition to CXR and US. 47 consecutive cases of occult PTX (on CXR) were evaluated and compared with controls. Three signs were evaluated: lung sliding, the A-line sign, and the lung point. The abolition of lung sliding alone had sensitivity of 100% and specificity of 78%. Absent lung sliding plus the A-line sign had sensitivity of 95% and specificity of 94%. The lung point had sensitivity and specificity of 79% and 100%, respectively	ICU study on occult PTX. It is critical to diagnose PTX in this patient population because of the risk of converting to tension PTX on ventilators with positive pressure
Volpicelli,[68] 2011	Evidence-based and expert consensus recommendations for lung US in critical care and emergency settings. A literature review of 320 references was performed, as well as expert recommendations from a multidisciplinary panel of 28 experts from 8 countries	Outstanding analysis, and key recommendations and levels of evidence regarding all aspects of point-of-care lung US (including trauma)
Alrajhi et al,[69] 2012	570 articles were reviewed and 21 selected for full review. Of these, 8 studies met criteria. All studies but one used lung sliding and comet tailing to rule out PTX. A total of 1048 patients were included. US was 90.9% sensitive and 98.2% specific for the detection of PTX, compared with CXR (50.2% sensitivity and 99.4% specificity)	Meta-analysis confirming excellent sensitivity and specificity of lung US primarily utilizing the lung-sliding and comet-tail signs

Abbreviations: AP, anteroposterior; CT, computed tomography; CXR, chest radiography; ED, emergency department; ICU, intensive care unit; PTX, pneumothorax; US, ultrasonography.

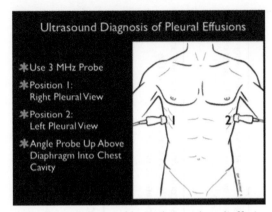

Fig. 21. Probe placement for evaluation of hemothorax/pleural effusion.

- Hemothorax evaluation is performed with the 3- to 5-MHz probe during the diaphragmatic evaluation of the RUQ and LUQ as discussed earlier (**Figs. 21 and 22**).
- Pneumothorax evaluation is best performed with a high-frequency linear probe (≥10 MHz).
- Technique (see also the article on thoracic aspects elsewhere in this issue)
  a. Right chest: Assess for pneumothorax on the right by placing the probe in a longitudinal orientation (indicator marker toward head) in the second intercostal space along the midclavicular line. With high clinical suspicion, scan through other parts of the chest (**Figs. 23–25**).
  b. Evaluate for presence or absence of lung sliding (a real-time appearance of shimmering at the pleural line that has the appearance of ants walking across the screen). Lung sliding is absent in the location of a pneumothorax.
  c. Evaluate for comet-tail artifact (short vertical lines emanating off the pleural line, **Fig. 26**). Comet-tail artifact is absent in the location of a pneumothorax.

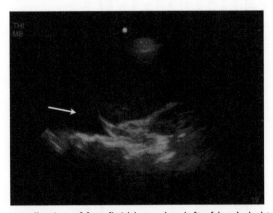

Fig. 22. Hemothorax: collection of free fluid (*arrow*) to left of (cephalad to) the diaphragm.

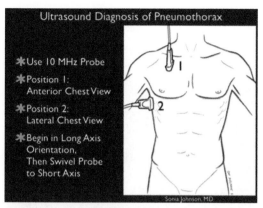

Fig. 23. Probe placement for pneumothorax evaluation.

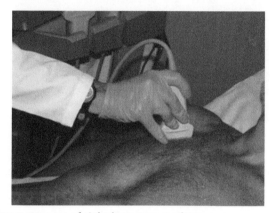

Fig. 24. Probe placement: scan of right lung pneumothorax.

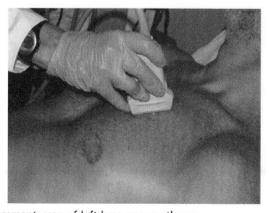

Fig. 25. Probe placement: scan of left lung pneumothorax.

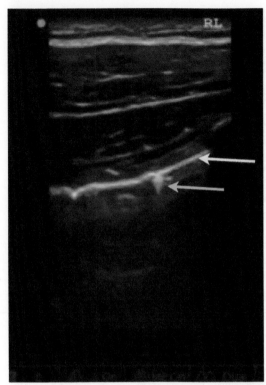

Fig. 26. Short vertical comet tails (*blue arrow*) emanating from pleural line (*yellow arrow*).

d. The "sandy beach" appearance on M-mode scanning can also confirm absence of pneumothorax; conversely, the "stratosphere sign" or "barcode sign" indicates the presence of pneumothorax (**Figs. 27** and **28**).
e. Left chest: Repeat as above, on the left side.
f. If identified, the "lung point" shows the edge of the pneumothorax, where lung sliding abruptly ends.

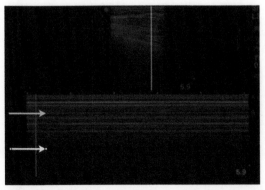

Fig. 27. "Sandy beach" sign of normal lung on M-mode. The "waves" (*blue arrow*) lay above the "sand" (*yellow arrow*).

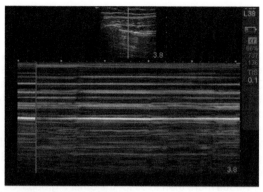

Fig. 28. "Stratosphere sign" of pneumothorax.

STATE OF FAST, 2013: CONTROVERSIES

This article aims to provide an evidence-based review of both the strengths and limitations of the FAST examination in adults. Despite the plethora of evidence supporting the utility of the FAST, there continues to be ongoing debate. Awareness of these continuing issues is imperative if interdisciplinary trauma protocols that optimize patient outcomes in a rational, resource-efficient manner are to be developed.

Melniker and colleagues[70] performed a randomized, controlled clinical trial evaluating the time from ED arrival to transfer to operative care in patients with torso trauma, with the intervention being incorporation of a point-of-care limited sonography (PLUS) protocol versus usual care. Secondary outcomes included CT use, length of stay, complications, and charges. There were no important differences in the characteristics of the groups, and both groups included both stable and unstable patients. Compared with the usual-care group, time to operative care was 64% less for PLUS patients. PLUS patients also underwent fewer CT scans (odds ratio 0.16), spent 27% fewer days in the hospital, and had fewer complications (odds ratio 0.16). Charges were 35% less in comparison with controls. This important study showed that ultrasonography enhanced care and efficiency, all at a lower cost.

A Cochrane database review of the FAST caused concern when it suggested that evidence from randomized controlled trials was insufficient to justify promotion of ultrasonography-based clinical pathways in diagnosing patients with suspected blunt abdominal trauma.[71] However, this study included only 4 articles, 2 of which showed more rapid/efficient care provided with the FAST examination.[72] In addition, when this review was further analyzed, questions arose as to its methodology and suggested that it was flawed.[73]

Natarajan and colleagues[74] posed the question of whether the FAST scan is worth doing in patients with hemodynamically stable blunt trauma. A total of 2105 patients with blunt trauma were evaluated, and 1894 true-negative studies were performed (1201 confirmed with CT and the rest with observation). 88 true-positive studies and 118 false negatives were found. Of the false negatives, 44 eventually required laparotomy. Natarajan and colleagues[74] suggest that the FAST scan should be reserved for hemodynamically unstable patients. However, their own results speak against this. The investigators were able to identify 88 patients with a positive FAST before they became hemodynamically unstable; they avoided CT imaging in 693 patients with negative FAST scans who were evaluated with observation alone after their negative FAST, and only 2% of all of their negative FAST scans needed to go to the operating room (OR).

In 2009, Melniker[75] published a rebuttal to the controversial Cochrane review. In his study, he performed a systematic literature review using verbatim methodologies as described in the Cochrane review with the exception of telephone contacts. Of 487 citations, 163 articles were fully screened, and 11 contained prospectively derived data (instead of the 4 articles cited by Cochrane). Of the 2755 patients in these studies, 16% went to the OR after FAST. Based on this extensive review, Melniker concluded that the FAST examination, when adequately completed, is a nearly perfect test for predicting a "need for OR" in patients with blunt torso trauma.[75]

Becker and colleagues[76] evaluated the reliability of the FAST scan in patients with a high injury severity score (ISS). In their study, 3181 blunt abdominal trauma patients were split into 3 groups based on ISS (groups 1, 2, and 3 with ISS means of 7.9, 19.6, and 41.3, respectively). The accuracy of ultrasonography was 90.6% in the most injured group, versus more than 97% for the other 2 groups. Severely injured patients benefited greatly from early ultrasonographic detection of hemodynamically significant injuries.

In summary, it is clear that despite the controversy, the evidence overwhelmingly supports the recommendation to take unstable adult patients with a positive FAST to the OR. Patients with a negative FAST require further evaluation, with serial examinations, laboratory tests, or imaging, depending on the clinical presentation and management options available.

FUTURE DIRECTIONS
Pulseless Traumatic Arrest

The cardiac views of the E-FAST examination can provide very useful information during the initial resuscitation of a trauma patient. An important study by Cureton and colleagues[77] in 2012 discussed the utility of the cardiac portion of the FAST in pulseless traumatic arrest. To date this is the largest study published on this important topic, being a retrospective analysis of 318 adult trauma patients who were pulseless on hospital arrival. Electrocardiograms and cardiac ultrasonography were performed on 162 of these patients. The sensitivity of cardiac motion on ultrasonography to predict survival to admission was 86%, with a negative predictive value of 99%. This result suggests that the cardiac view of the E-FAST examination may be a rapid method to determine the futility of resuscitation in this patient group, although further studies are warranted. The reader is referred to the articles on echo and resuscitation elsewhere in this issue for a further discussion on future directions of trauma echo.

Contrast-Enhanced Ultrasonography for Solid-Organ Injury

One of the weaknesses of ultrasonography is its inability to effectively evaluate solid-organ injury. Contrast-enhanced ultrasonography, if available, may be beneficial in these cases.[78] Blaivas and colleagues[79] studied the feasibility of using intravenous contrast during the FAST examination in simulated patients. The mean time to initial visualization of contrast was 15 seconds; the latent phase of the intravenous contrast occurred at a mean time of 54 seconds. It was postulated that contrast enhancement would allow better ultrasonographic visualization of hematomas that were not actively bleeding.

Chest-Tube Placement

The utility of ultrasonography in diagnosing hemothoraces and pneumothoraces has been well studied. Bedside ultrasonography has also been shown to be valuable in the management of chest tubes. Ultrasound-guided intercostal nerve blocks can decrease the pain associated with chest-tube placement.[80] In addition, intrathoracic chest-tube placement can be confirmed with ultrasonography.[81]

Diagnosis of Pelvic Fracture

Regarding the limitations of diagnosing hemorrhage from a pelvic-fracture source (as discussed earlier), ultrasonography has shown some utility in the diagnosis of pubic symphysis widening suggestive of unstable pelvic fractures. This modality could potentially lead to faster application of a pelvic binder and tamponade of bleeding,[82] especially if there was a delay in obtaining the pelvic radiograph.

Hemodynamic Evaluation

The FAST examination has been incorporated into the Rapid Ultrasound in Shock Protocol, a targeted assessment for the rapid diagnosis of the etiology of undifferentiated hypotension. It is also a major component of the CORE scan (a Concentrated Overview of Resuscitative Efforts). Changes in the IVC diameter correlate directly with intravascular volume status.[83] A flat IVC (less than 2 cm) has been shown to be an indicator of poor prognosis in trauma patients and acute surgical patients.[84] The IVC is normally assessed in the subxiphoid view, but can also be visualized using a midaxillary view. This view may be more easily obtained in patients with abdominal pain, and is obtained with the probe in the same position as the RUQ FAST view by fanning anteriorly.[85] Serial IVC measurements can be used to help guide intravascular volume resuscitation.

Prehospital, Mass Casualty, and Practice in Austere Environments

Many countries are now incorporating the E-FAST examination into prehospital protocols, as it has the potential to significantly affect scene management. In Europe, physicians routinely ride along in ambulances. A recent study shows promise in utilizing ultrasonography in the periarrest setting. Echo findings altered management in 78% of these cases.[86] Although these systems differ from those in the United States, early studies show promise in the ability to teach basic elements of the E-FAST to paramedics in the United States.[87] However, care must be taken to ensure the appropriate balance of scene time to optimize survival.

With its beginnings in the Armenian earthquake mass casualty incident (MCI), ultrasonography continues to have significant utility in MCIs such as the Haiti earthquake, for both trauma evaluation and venous access.[55,88] In fact, new ultrasonography protocols are being developed that take advantage of the portable nature of this modality during MCIs.

The CAVEAT examination by Stawicki and colleagues[89] incorporates the well-established abdominal and thoracic applications discussed here, as well as assessment for long-bone fractures. Ultrasonography has tremendous potential in multiple extreme environments, even including the International Space Station.[90]

There were 5.1 million deaths from injury worldwide in 2010.[1] Expanding the use of point-of-care ultrasonography in the global care of trauma patients, especially to those in resource-limited areas, has the potential to have a massive impact on mortality.

SUMMARY

The E-FAST evaluation provides critical information during the real-time evaluation of complex trauma patients. It can identify free fluid suggestive of abdominal solid-organ injury, hemothorax, or pericardial fluid collections. Its sensitivity for pneumothorax is superior to that of CXR.

This article reviews important literature on the FAST and E-FAST examinations in the acute care setting. Also reviewed are key pitfalls, limitations, and controversies. A practical "how-to" guide and exploration of new frontiers are presented. The authors hope that this knowledge will enable physicians and their teams to further optimize trauma care, both in the United States and abroad.

REFERENCES

1. Lozano R, Naghavi M, Foreman K, et al. Global and regional mortality from 235 causes of death for 20 age groups in 1990 and 2010: a systematic analysis for the Global Burden of Disease Study 2010. Lancet 2013;380(9859):2095–128.
2. US Department of Transportation National Highway Traffic Safety Administration, A Brief Statistical Summary. Early estimate of motor vehicle traffic fatalities for the first nine months (January-September) of 2012. Vol. December 2012; 2012. Available at: www.nrd.nhtsa.dot.gov/Pubs/811706.pdf.
3. Centers for Disease Control and Prevention (CDC). Years of potential life lost from unintentional injuries among persons aged 0-19 years-United States, 2000-2009. MMWR Morb Mortal Wkly Rep 2012;61(41):830–3.
4. Karch DL, Logan J, McDaniel D, et al. Surveillance for violent deaths—National Violent Death Reporting System, 16 states, 2009. MMWR Surveill Summ 2012;61(6):1–43.
5. Centers for Disease Control and Prevention. Injury prevention and control 2012. Available at: http://www.cdc.gov/injury/overview/leading_cod.html. Accessed January 8, 2013.
6. Institute of Medicine Committee on the Future of Emergency Care in the U.S. Health System. The future of emergency care in the United States health system. Ann Emerg Med 2006;48(2):115–20.
7. ACEP Policy Statement. Emergency Ultrasound Guidelines. Annals of Emerg Med 2009;53:550–70.
8. AIUM officially recognizes ACEP emergency ultrasound guidelines. 2011. Available at: http://www.acep.org/News-Media-top-banner/AIUM-Officially-Recognizes-ACEP-Emergency-Ultrasound-Guidelines/. Accessed January 3, 2013.
9. American College of Surgeons Committee on Trauma. Advanced Trauma Life Support® (ATLS®). 9th edition. Chicago (IL): American College of Surgeons; 2012.
10. Rozycki GS, Root HD. The diagnosis of intraabdominal visceral injury. J Trauma 2010;68(5):1019–23.
11. Moore CL, Copel JA. Point-of-care ultrasonography. N Engl J Med 2011;364(8): 749–57.
12. Hoff WS, Holevar M, Nagy KK, et al. Practice management guidelines for the evaluation of blunt abdominal trauma: the East Practice Management Guidelines Work Group. J Trauma 2002;53(3):602–15.
13. Rodriguez A, DuPriest RW Jr, Shatney CH. Recognition of intra-abdominal injury in blunt trauma victims. A prospective study comparing physical examination with peritoneal lavage. Am Surg 1982;48(9):457–9.
14. Schurink GW, Bode PJ, van Luijt PA, et al. The value of physical examination in the diagnosis of patients with blunt abdominal trauma: a retrospective study. Injury 1997;28(4):261–5.
15. Kirkpatrick AW. Clinician-performed focused sonography for the resuscitation of trauma. Crit Care Med 2007;35(Suppl 5):S162–72.
16. Melanson SW. The FAST Exam: a review of the literature. In: Jehle D, Heller MB, editors. Ultrasonography in trauma: the FAST Exam. Dallas (TX): American College of Emergency Physicians; 2003. p. 127–45.

17. Jehle D, Guarino J, Karamanoukian H. Emergency department ultrasound in the evaluation of blunt abdominal trauma. Am J Emerg Med 1993;11(4):342–6.
18. Rothlin MA, Naf R, Amgwerd M, et al. Ultrasound in blunt abdominal and thoracic trauma. J Trauma 1993;34(4):488–95.
19. Rozycki GS, Ochsner MG, Schmidt JA, et al. A prospective study of surgeon-performed ultrasound as the primary adjuvant modality for injured patient assessment. J Trauma 1995;39(3):492–8 [discussion: 498–500].
20. Ma OJ, Mateer JR. Trauma ultrasound examination versus chest radiography in the detection of hemothorax. Ann Emerg Med 1997;29(3):312–5 [discussion: 315–6].
21. Brooks A, Davies B, Smethhurst M, et al. Emergency ultrasound in the acute assessment of haemothorax. Emerg Med J 2004;21(1):44–6.
22. Lee BC, Ormsby EL, McGahan JP, et al. The utility of sonography for the triage of blunt abdominal trauma patients to exploratory laparotomy. AJR Am J Roentgenol 2007;188(2):415–21.
23. Stengel D, Bauwens K, Rademacher G, et al. Association between compliance with methodological standards of diagnostic research and reported test accuracy: meta-analysis of focused assessment of US for trauma. Radiology 2005; 236(1):102–11.
24. Quinn AC, Sinert R. What is the utility of the Focused Assessment with Sonography in Trauma (FAST) exam in penetrating torso trauma? Injury 2011;42(5): 482–7.
25. Rozycki GS, Ballard RB, Feliciano DV, et al. Surgeon-performed ultrasound for the assessment of truncal injuries: lessons learned from 1540 patients. Ann Surg 1998;228(4):557–67.
26. Plummer D, Brunette D, Asinger R, et al. Emergency department echocardiography improves outcome in penetrating cardiac injury. Ann Emerg Med 1992; 21(6):709–12.
27. Wherrett LJ, Boulanger BR, McLellan BA, et al. Hypotension after blunt abdominal trauma: the role of emergent abdominal sonography in surgical triage. J Trauma 1996;41(5):815–20.
28. Rozycki GS, Feliciano DV, Ochsner MG, et al. The role of ultrasound in patients with possible penetrating cardiac wounds: a prospective multicenter study. J Trauma 1999;46(4):543–51 [discussion: 551–2].
29. Rose JS, Richards JR, Battistella F, et al. The fast is positive, now what? Derivation of a clinical decision rule to determine the need for therapeutic laparotomy in adults with blunt torso trauma and a positive trauma ultrasound. J Emerg Med 2005;29(1):15–21.
30. Boulanger BR, McLellan BA, Brenneman FD, et al. Emergent abdominal sonography as a screening test in a new diagnostic algorithm for blunt trauma. J Trauma 1996;40(6):867–74.
31. Boulanger BR, Brenneman FD, McLellan BA, et al. A prospective study of emergent abdominal sonography after blunt trauma. J Trauma 1995;39(2):325–30.
32. Ma OJ, Kefer MP, Mateer JR, et al. Evaluation of hemoperitoneum using a single-vs multiple-view ultrasonographic examination. Acad Emerg Med 1995;2(7): 581–6.
33. Healey MA, Simons RK, Winchell RJ, et al. A prospective evaluation of abdominal ultrasound in blunt trauma: is it useful? J Trauma 1996;40(6):875–83 [discussion: 883–5].
34. Blackbourne LH, Soffer D, McKenney M, et al. Secondary ultrasound examination increases the sensitivity of the FAST exam in blunt trauma. J Trauma 2004; 57(5):934–8.

35. Shackford SR, Rogers FB, Osler TM, et al. Focused abdominal sonogram for trauma: the learning curve of nonradiologist clinicians in detecting hemoperitoneum. J Trauma 1999;46(4):553–62 [discussion: 562–4].

36. Jang T, Kryder G, Sineff S, et al. The technical errors of physicians learning to perform focused assessment with sonography in trauma. Acad Emerg Med 2012;19(1):98–101.

37. Branney SW, Wolfe RE, Moore EE, et al. Quantitative sensitivity of ultrasound in detecting free intraperitoneal fluid. J Trauma 1995;39(2):375–80.

38. Von Kuenssberg Jehle D, Stiller G, Wagner D. Sensitivity in detecting free intraperitoneal fluid with the pelvic views of the FAST exam. Am J Emerg Med 2003; 21(6):476–8.

39. Brownstein MR, Bunting T, Meyer AA, et al. Diagnosis and management of blunt small bowel injury: a survey of the membership of the American Association for the Surgery of Trauma. J Trauma 2000;48(3):402–7.

40. Banz VM, Butt MU, Zimmermann H, et al. Free abdominal fluid without obvious solid organ injury upon CT imaging: an actual problem or simply over-diagnosing? J Trauma Manag Outcomes 2009;3:10.

41. Korner M, Krotz MM, Degenhart C, et al. Current role of emergency US in patients with major trauma. Radiographics 2008;28(1):225–42.

42. McGahan JP, Richards J, Fogata ML. Emergency ultrasound in trauma patients. Radiol Clin North Am 2004;42(2):417–25.

43. Brown MA, Casola G, Sirlin CB, et al. Importance of evaluating organ parenchyma during screening abdominal ultrasonography after blunt trauma. J Ultrasound Med 2001;20(6):577–83 [quiz: 585].

44. Schnuriger B, Kilz J, Inderbitzin D, et al. The accuracy of FAST in relation to grade of solid organ injuries: a retrospective analysis of 226 trauma patients with liver or splenic lesion. BMC Med Imaging 2009;9:3.

45. Tayal VS, Nielsen A, Jones AE, et al. Accuracy of trauma ultrasound in major pelvic injury. J Trauma 2006;61(6):1453–7.

46. Friese RS, Malekzadeh S, Shafi S, et al. Abdominal ultrasound is an unreliable modality for the detection of hemoperitoneum in patients with pelvic fracture. J Trauma 2007;63(1):97–102.

47. Ballard RB, Rozycki GS, Newman PG, et al. An algorithm to reduce the incidence of false-negative FAST examinations in patients at high risk for occult injury. Focused Assessment for the Sonographic Examination of the Trauma patient. J Am Coll Surg 1999;189(2):145–50 [discussion: 150–1].

48. Kuncir EJ, Velmahos GC. Diagnostic peritoneal aspiration—the foster child of DPL: a prospective observational study. Int J Surg 2007;5(3):167–71.

49. Kendall JL, Ramos JP. Fluid-filled bowel mimicking hemoperitoneum: a false-positive finding during sonographic evaluation for trauma. J Emerg Med 2003; 25(1):79–82.

50. Sierzenski PR, Schofer JM, Bauman MJ, et al. The double-line sign: a false positive finding on the Focused Assessment with Sonography for Trauma (FAST) examination. J Emerg Med 2011;40(2):188–9.

51. Laselle BT, Byyny RL, Haukoos JS, et al. False-negative FAST examination: associations with injury characteristics and patient outcomes. Ann Emerg Med 2012;60(3):326–34.e3.

52. Peitzman AB, Harbrecht BG, Rivera L, et al. Failure of observation of blunt splenic injury in adults: variability in practice and adverse consequences. J Am Coll Surg 2005;201(2):179–87.

53. Sirlin CB, Brown MA, Andrade-Barreto OA, et al. Blunt abdominal trauma: clinical value of negative screening US scans. Radiology 2004;230(3): 661–8.

54. Branney SW, Moore EE, Cantrill SV, et al. Ultrasound based key clinical pathway reduces the use of hospital resources for the evaluation of blunt abdominal trauma. J Trauma 1997;42(6):1086–90.

55. Sarkisian AE, Khondkarian RA, Amirbekian NM, et al. Sonographic screening of mass casualties for abdominal and renal injuries following the 1988 Armenian earthquake. J Trauma 1991;31(2):247–50.

56. Nishijima DK, Simel DL, Wisner DH, et al. Does this adult patient have a blunt intra-abdominal injury? JAMA 2012;307(14):1517–27.

57. Chambers JA, Pilbrow WJ. Ultrasound in abdominal trauma: an alternative to peritoneal lavage. Arch Emerg Med 1988;5(1):26–33.

58. Abrams BJ, Sukumvanich P, Seibel R, et al. Ultrasound for the detection of intra-peritoneal fluid: the role of Trendelenburg positioning. Am J Emerg Med 1999; 17(2):117–20.

59. Zanobetti M, Poggioni C, Pini R. Can chest ultrasonography replace standard chest radiography for evaluation of acute dyspnea in the ED? Chest 2011; 139(5):1140–7.

60. Ball CG, Kirkpatrick AW, Feliciano DV. The occult pneumothorax: what have we learned? Can J Surg 2009;52(5):E173–9.

61. Blaivas M, Lyon M, Duggal S. A prospective comparison of supine chest radiography and bedside ultrasound for the diagnosis of traumatic pneumothorax. Acad Emerg Med 2005;12(9):844–9.

62. Kirkpatrick AW, Sirois M, Laupland KB, et al. Hand-held thoracic sonography for detecting post-traumatic pneumothoraces: the Extended Focused Assessment with Sonography for Trauma (EFAST). J Trauma 2004;57(2):288–95.

63. Lichtenstein DA, Meziere G, Lascols N, et al. Ultrasound diagnosis of occult pneumothorax. Crit Care Med 2005;33(6):1231–8.

64. Goodman TR, Traill ZC, Phillips AJ, et al. Ultrasound detection of pneumothorax. Clin Radiol 1999;54(11):736–9.

65. Abboud PA, Kendall J. Emergency department ultrasound for hemothorax after blunt traumatic injury. J Emerg Med 2003;25(2):181–4.

66. Ball CG, Ranson K, Dente CJ, et al. Clinical predictors of occult pneumothoraces in severely injured blunt polytrauma patients: a prospective observational study. Injury 2009;40(1):44–7.

67. Volpicelli G, Elbarbary M, Blaivas M, et al. International evidence-based recommendations for point-of-care lung ultrasound. Intensive Care Med 2012;38(4): 577–91.

68. Volpicelli G. Sonographic diagnosis of pneumothorax. Intensive Care Med 2011; 37(2):224–32.

69. Alrajhi K, Woo MY, Vaillancourt C. Test characteristics of ultrasonography for the detection of pneumothorax: a systematic review and meta-analysis. Chest 2012; 141(3):703–8.

70. Melniker LA, Leibner E, McKenney MG, et al. Randomized controlled clinical trial of point-of-care, limited ultrasonography for trauma in the emergency department: the first sonography outcomes assessment program trial. Ann Emerg Med 2006;48(3):227–35.

71. Stengel D, Bauwens K, Sehouli J, et al. Emergency ultrasound-based algorithms for diagnosing blunt abdominal trauma. Cochrane Database Syst Rev 2005;(2):CD004446.

72. Vance S. Evidence-based emergency medicine/systematic review abstract. The FAST scan: are we improving care of the trauma patient? Ann Emerg Med 2007; 49(3):364–6.

73. Hosek WT, McCarthy ML. Trauma ultrasound and the 2005 Cochrane Review. Ann Emerg Med 2007;50(5):619–20 [author reply: 620–1]; [discussion: 621].

74. Natarajan B, Gupta PK, Cemaj S, et al. FAST scan: is it worth doing in hemodynamically stable blunt trauma patients? Surgery 2010;148(4):695–700 [discussion: 700–1].

75. Melniker L. The value of focused assessment with sonography in trauma examination for the need for operative intervention in blunt torso trauma: a rebuttal to "emergency ultrasound-based algorithms for diagnosing blunt abdominal trauma (review)", from the Cochrane Collaboration. Crit Ultrasound J 2009;1:73–84.

76. Becker A, Lin G, McKenney MG, et al. Is the FAST exam reliable in severely injured patients? Injury 2010;41(5):479–83.

77. Cureton EL, Yeung LY, Kwan RO, et al. The heart of the matter: utility of ultrasound of cardiac activity during traumatic arrest. J Trauma Acute Care Surg 2012;73(1):102–10.

78. Valentino M, Serra C, Pavlica P, et al. Contrast-enhanced ultrasound for blunt abdominal trauma. Semin Ultrasound CT MR 2007;28(2):130–40.

79. Blaivas M, Lyon M, Brannam L, et al. Feasibility of FAST examination performance with ultrasound contrast. J Emerg Med 2005;29(3):307–11.

80. Stone MB, Carnell J, Fischer JW, et al. Ultrasound-guided intercostal nerve block for traumatic pneumothorax requiring tube thoracostomy. Am J Emerg Med 2011;29(6):697.e1–2.

81. Jenkins JA, Gharahbaghian L, Doniger SJ, et al. Sonographic Identification of Tube Thoracostomy Study (SITTS): confirmation of intrathoracic placement. West J Emerg Med 2012;13(4):305–11.

82. Bauman M, Marinaro J, Tawil I, et al. Ultrasonographic determination of pubic symphyseal widening in trauma: the FAST-PS study. J Emerg Med 2011;40(5): 528–33.

83. Perera P, Mailhot T, Riley D, et al. The RUSH exam: rapid ultrasound in shock in the evaluation of the critically ill. Emerg Med Clin North Am 2010;28(1):29–56, vii.

84. Ferrada P, Vanguri P, Anand RJ, et al. Flat inferior vena cava: indicator of poor prognosis in trauma and acute care surgery patients. Am Surg 2012;78(12): 1396–8.

85. Howard ZD, Gharahbaghian L, Steele BJ, et al. Midaxillary Option for Measuring IVC (MOMI): prospective comparison of the right midaxillary and subxiphoid IVC. Measurements Ann Emerg Med 2012;60(4):S78–9.

86. Testa A, Cibinel GA, Portale G, et al. The proposal of an integrated ultrasonographic approach into the ALS algorithm for cardiac arrest: the PEA protocol. Eur Rev Med Pharmacol Sci 2010;14(2):77–88.

87. Chin EJ, Chan CH, Mortazavi R, et al. A pilot study examining the viability of a Prehospital Assessment with UltraSound for Emergencies (PAUSE) protocol. J Emerg Med 2013;44(1):142–9.

88. Shorter M, Macias DJ. Portable handheld ultrasound in austere environments: use in the Haiti disaster. Prehospital Disaster Med 2012;27(2):172–7.

89. Stawicki SP, Howard JM, Pryor JP, et al. Portable ultrasonography in mass casualty incidents: the CAVEAT examination. World J Orthop 2010;1(1):10–9.

90. Ma OJ, Norvell JG, Subramanian S. Ultrasound applications in mass casualties and extreme environments. Crit Care Med 2007;35(Suppl 5):S275–9.

The CORE Scan
Concentrated Overview of Resuscitative Efforts

Teresa S. Wu, MD

KEYWORDS

- Resuscitation ultrasound • CORE scan • Emergency bedside ultrasonography

KEY POINTS

- Ultrasound can be used at the patient's bedside to make critical diagnoses that can help expedite and improve patient care.
- During a critical resuscitation, the CORE scan can be used to identify life-threatening causes for a patient's deterioration and help guide management options.
- Emergent procedures can be performed under ultrasound guidance during resuscitation attempts.
- The CORE scan can be repeated if serial exams are required.

INTRODUCTION

Critically ill patients require rapid, accurate assessments and appropriate therapeutic interventions to maximize their chances of recovery. Often, the cause of a patient's decompensation is not readily apparent based solely on history and physical examination findings. Furthermore, the evaluation of resuscitation efforts is often difficult because of the time-intensive and invasive nature of most monitoring techniques. The use of bedside ultrasonography has been successfully integrated universally into the assessment of patients presenting with acute traumatic injury.[1,2] Various protocols are also being studied regarding the use of bedside ultrasonography in the evaluation of patients presenting with shock and undifferentiated hypotension, and during volume resuscitation.[3–6] This article describes a compendium of bedside scans that should be performed during the assessment and management of critically ill patients. The CORE (Concentrated Overview of Resuscitative Efforts) scan can be used to help make critical diagnoses and guide resuscitation efforts in patients with undifferentiated deterioration.

ENDOTRACHEAL TUBE ASSESSMENT

The first part of the CORE scan addresses the patient's airway. Traditionally, assessment of proper endotracheal tube placement has been performed using methods such

EM Residency Program, Department of Emergency Medicine, Maricopa Medical Center, University of Arizona, College of Medicine-Phoenix, 2601 East Roosevelt Street, Phoenix, AZ 85008, USA
E-mail address: teresawumd@gmail.com

Crit Care Clin 30 (2014) 151–175
http://dx.doi.org/10.1016/j.ccc.2013.08.001   criticalcare.theclinics.com

as direct laryngoscopy, auscultation of breath sounds, end-tidal CO_2 detection, and chest radiography. Ultrasonography has been shown to be useful in determining proper endotracheal tube positioning at the bedside.[7] During intubation attempts, a linear-array transducer can be placed in a horizontal fashion across the patient's neck, at the level of the cricothyroid membrane. The orientation marker on the probe is typically oriented toward the patient's right (**Fig. 1**).

With the probe in this position, the patient's thyroid can be visualized nearfield on the screen, with the bright white hyperechoic rings of the trachea just farfield to it (**Fig. 2**).

As the endotracheal tube is being passed down through the trachea, the bright white hyperechoic tube can be visualized entering the tracheal lumen. The tube will cast a white acoustic shadow farfield on the screen once it is in the lumen of the trachea (**Fig. 3**).

On ultrasonography, the esophagus can be seen as a muscular ring just postero-lateral to the trachea. During the intubation, applying color Doppler over the trachea can help visualize movement of the endotracheal tube as it is advanced into the trachea (**Fig. 4**).

If the endotracheal tube is accidentally passed into the esophagus, the comet tails from the tube will be seen in the esophagus, and a flash of color will be seen on color Doppler imaging of the esophagus during the failed intubation attempt (**Fig. 5**).

Endotracheal ultrasonography can be useful in guiding proper tube placement during the initial intubation attempt, or for reassessment of tube placement following patient transfer, repositioning, or changes in a patient's respiratory status. Performing bedside ultrasonography to determine tube positioning is faster than performing a direct laryngoscopy, and carries less risk of accidentally dislodging the endotracheal tube. Once the endotracheal tube has been confirmed to be properly in the trachea, it is useful to evaluate the lungs for symmetric, bilateral lung inflation and lung sliding during ventilation and oxygenation attempts.

BEDSIDE PULMONARY ULTRASONOGRAPHY

The CORE scan can be modified based on the clinical suspicion of what is likely contributing to a patient's deterioration. In most situations, once the endotracheal tube position has been confirmed within the trachea, it is useful to evaluate the lungs as the next step. A thoracic ultrasonographic scan can be completed quickly at the

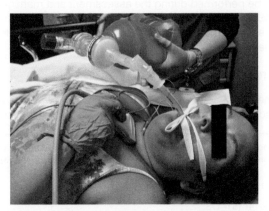

Fig. 1. Ultrasonographic evaluation of endotracheal tube placement. Note that the indicator marker should be directed toward the patient's right side.

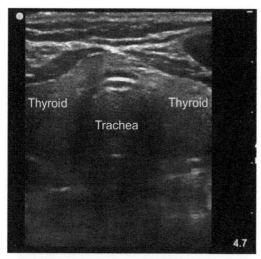

Fig. 2. Ultrasonographic visualization of the hyperechoic tracheal rings and empty trachea behind the thyroid tissue.

bedside to determine whether the patient has ventilation of both lungs and to assess whether the patient has a pneumothorax or pleural effusion that needs to be emergently addressed.

The lungs can be visualized by placing either a high-frequency linear-array transducer or a lower-frequency curvilinear transducer in a horizontal fashion in the second or third intercostal space (**Fig. 6**).

With the probe in this position, the parietal and visceral pleural interface can be seen as a bright white hyperechoic line coursing horizontally across the ultrasound screen.

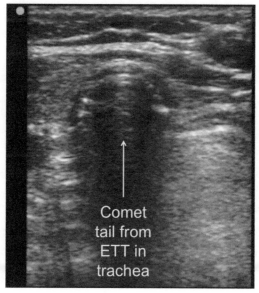

Fig. 3. Endotracheal tube within the tracheal lumen producing a hyperechoic comet-tail farfield.

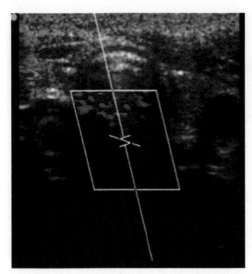

Fig. 4. Improving visualization of the endotracheal tube entering the trachea using color Doppler.

For patients in whom it is difficult to identify the pleural line, begin the scan with the probe in a longitudinal fashion, at the third intercostal space, along the midclavicular line; this will provide a view of the ribs and underlying structures. To ensure proper visualization of the parietal-visceral pleural interface, locate an anechoic rib and focus on the hyperechoic line just farfield to the rib (**Fig. 7**).

During the normal inspiratory and expiratory cycle, the visceral pleura can be seen gliding along the parietal pleura. On ultrasonography, this horizontal to-and-fro movement across the screen has been termed lung sliding.[8] If a patient is intubated with the endotracheal tube in the proper position, bagging the patient should produce bilateral lung sliding with each ventilation. If the endotracheal tube is in the right mainstem bronchus, there will be an absence of lung sliding on the left. Similarly, with

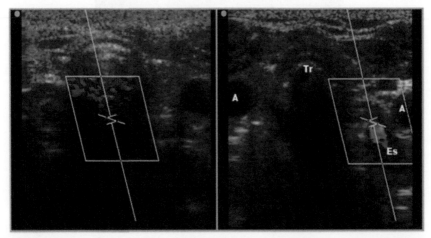

Fig. 5. Comparison of color Doppler imaging of the endotracheal tube entering the trachea (*left*) versus the esophagus (*right*). A, carotid artery; Es, esophagus; Tr, tracheal rings.

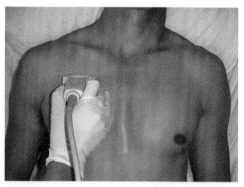

Fig. 6. Linear array transducer and probe placement for a thoracic ultrasound.

an endobronchial intubation on the left, lung sliding will not be seen over the right hemithorax.

If lung sliding is difficult to visualize, or if a unilateral pneumothorax is suspected, the next step is to evaluate the diaphragm for bilateral, symmetric excursion. The diaphragm is best visualized by placing a lower-frequency curvilinear or phased-array transducer in a longitudinal fashion along the midaxillary line at the T7-T9 intercostal space (**Fig. 8**). With the indicator pointing toward the patient's head, the diaphragm will appear as a bright white hyperechoic line just to the left of the liver or the spleen (**Fig. 9**).

Compare the excursion of the diaphragm on both the left and right sides of the chest. If there is no lung sliding and no diaphragmatic excursion, the patient has an endobronchial mainstem intubation, a large unilateral airway obstruction, or a very large pneumothorax.

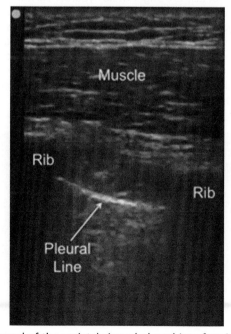

Fig. 7. Bedside ultrasound of the parietal-visceral pleural interface in between 2 anechoic ribs.

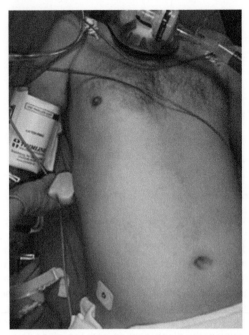

Fig. 8. Probe placement to evaluate the diaphragm for proper excursion during ventilation.

On ultrasonography, a normal lung typically demonstrates lung sliding and artifacts called comet tails. Comet tails are bright white hyperechoic artifacts that shoot farfield off the pleural interface when the parietal and visceral pleura appose one another during the respiratory cycle (**Fig. 10**). If there is air trapped in between the parietal and visceral pleura, comet tails and lung sliding will not be visualized.

When normal lung is visualized on M-mode, a characteristic pattern termed the seashore sign is seen (**Fig. 11**). The seashore sign depicts a normal interface between the lung and chest wall, where the static thoracic wall and soft tissue produces parallel lines across the screen. The pleural line is seen as a bright white horizontal line

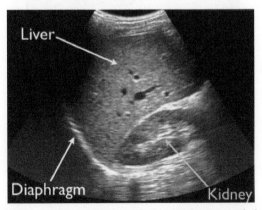

Fig. 9. Bedside ultrasonographic evaluation of the diaphragm and the inferior thoracic cavity.

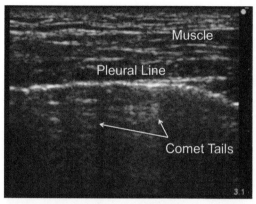

Fig. 10. Comet tails from a normal parietal-visceral pleural interface.

separating the soft tissue nearfield and the dynamic lung parenchyma farfield. If the patient has a pneumothorax, the M-mode imaging of the lung will produce a pattern called the stratosphere sign or bar-code sign (**Fig. 12**). This pattern is seen on M-mode because the air trapped in between the parietal and visceral pleura produces horizontal hyperechoic artifacts in the farfield.

If there is concern that there may be a pneumothorax instead of just an endobronchial mainstem intubation, scan along the chest until the edge of the pneumothorax is visualized. The transition point between normal lung and a pneumothorax is called the lung point.[9] At the lung point, normal lung sliding and comet tails will be seen abutting a region of the pleura where there is a distinct absence of lung sliding or comet tails. With B-mode scanning, it is easy to see the transition between the normal lung sliding across the screen and the stationary pneumothorax in real time (**Fig. 13**). On M-mode, if the cursor is placed directly over the lung point, a clear transition between the seashore sign and the bar-code sign will be observed (**Fig. 14**).

If thoracic ultrasonography does not demonstrate lung sliding and the lung point cannot be clearly visualized, it may be difficult to determine whether the patient has a pneumothorax or an endobronchial intubation. To help distinguish between the two entities, scan the lung for a lung pulse. The lung pulse is the detection of cardiac

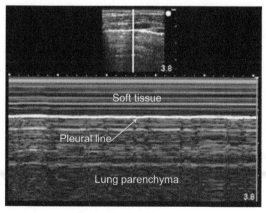

Fig. 11. The seashore sign: normal lung in M-mode.

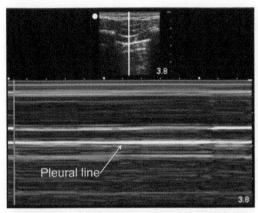

Fig. 12. The stratosphere sign or bar-code sign of a pneumothorax in M-mode.

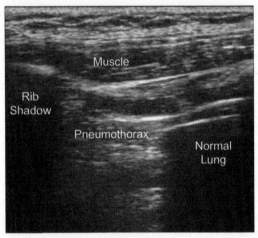

Fig. 13. A static image of the transition between normal lung and a pneumothorax at the lung point. In real-time B-mode scanning, the movement of the normal lung will be in distinct contrast to the stationary pneumothorax.

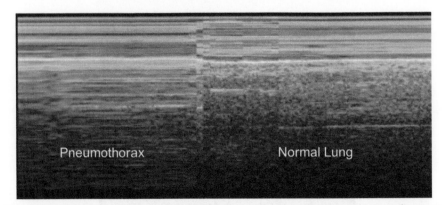

Fig. 14. Lung point on M-mode. Note the transition between the bar-code sign of a pneumothorax and the seashore sign of normal lung.

pulsations transmitted to the parietal pleura in a lung that is not being actively venti-lated, and is best visualized on M-mode. A lung pulse should not be visualized with a large pneumothorax. It is important to remember that lung sliding can be absent in patients who have had a pleurodesis, or who have pleural adhesions, pulmonary con-tusions, pulmonary infiltrates, acute respiratory distress syndrome, atelectasis, bullae, blebs, large pulmonary contusions, or pulmonary masses abutting the pleural line. Further research is being undertaken to help distinguish between these entities on bedside ultrasonography.

During the thoracic portion of the CORE scan, it is useful to know if the patient has a large pleural effusion that may require immediate intervention. Pleural effusions are best visualized by placing the probe in the mid- to posterior-axillary line between T7 and T10. Attempt to visualize the interface between the inferior lung and the dia-phragm. A pleural effusion will appear as a dark anechoic layer of fluid just cranial to the diaphragm. Lung may be seen floating in the effusion during the respiratory cycle (**Fig. 15**).

If the pleural effusion is thought to be contributing to the patient's deterioration, an emergent thoracostomy tube should be placed to drain the fluid noted on ultrasonography.

The CORE scan may demonstrate findings of pulmonary edema. Patients with clin-ically significant pulmonary edema will demonstrate large "B-lines" or "lung rockets" (**Fig. 16**). Lung rockets are bright white hyperechoic comet tails that move with sliding of the lung, and are the result of interlobular septa filled with water. These features are wider than the comet tails seen in normal lung, and should extend to the farfield depths of the ultrasound image. Patients with pulmonary edema should demonstrate more than two lung rockets in at least two areas of the thoracic cavity. Current research is under way to determine whether the number of lung rockets correlates with the degree of pulmonary edema. If lung rockets are visualized during the CORE scan, resuscitation and management options for alveolar-interstitial syndrome should be instituted accordingly.

BEDSIDE CARDIAC ULTRASONOGRAPHY

During the CORE scan, it is imperative to evaluate the heart to establish that the pa-tient still has cardiac activity; to note if there is a pericardial effusion and cardiac tam-ponade; to assess for any right ventricular strain that may indicate the presence of a

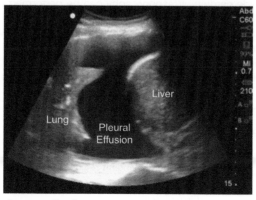

Fig. 15. Pleural effusion over the liver.

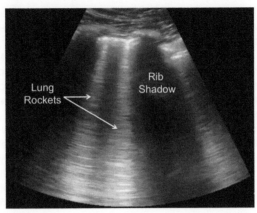

Fig. 16. "Lung rockets" from a patient with acute pulmonary edema.

large pulmonary embolism; to determine whether the patient requires more intravascular volume; and to evaluate the estimated ejection fraction of the heart.

To perform a rapid assessment of the heart during resuscitation attempts, it is ideal to start with a parasternal long-axis view of the heart. First, identify that the patient still has cardiac activity and that chest compressions are not warranted. Once cardiac activity has been visualized, assess for the presence of a pericardial effusion and cardiac tamponade. Pericardial fluid will appear as a dark anechoic stripe of fluid surrounding the heart. If the effusion is small, it may only be seen as a small black stripe of fluid along the posterior, dependent portion of the pericardial sac (**Table 1**). Larger effusions will be seen circumferentially around the heart and are typically more than 15 mm in diameter (**Fig. 17**).

The presence of a moderate or large pericardial effusion does not necessarily mean that the patient has cardiac tamponade. Ultrasonographic findings of cardiac tamponade include end-diastolic right ventricular collapse (**Fig. 18**), right atrial collapse, respiratory variation of blood flow across the tricuspid or mitral valve of more than 40%, and a dilated inferior vena cava (IVC) that does not change with inspiration or "sniffing" (**Fig. 19**).[10,11] If tamponade physiology is noted clinically or on bedside ultrasonography of the heart, a pericardiocentesis should be performed immediately under ultrasound guidance.[12]

If there is clinical suspicion for a large pulmonary embolism causing hemodynamic compromise, bedside cardiac ultrasonography can be performed to assess for right ventricular dilation (>1:1 right ventricular/left ventricular diameter) (**Fig. 20**), right ventricular systolic dysfunction, paradoxic septal bowing into the left ventricle (**Fig. 21**), IVC dilation without inspiratory collapse (**Fig. 22**), or presence of thrombus visualized in the right ventricle.[13] On a parasternal short-axis view of the heart, the septum may be seen bowing into the left ventricle, thereby creating the so-called D-sign from right

Table 1		
Categories of pericardial effusion		
Effusion Size	**Location**	**Diameter (mm)**
Small	Localized, dependent region	<10
Medium	Localized or circumferential	10–15
Large	Circumferential	>15

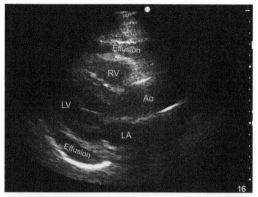

Fig. 17. Large pericardial effusion surrounding the heart. Ao, aortic outflow tract; LA, left atrium; LV, left ventricle; RV, right ventricle.

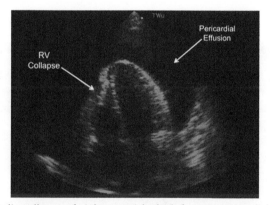

Fig. 18. End-diastolic collapse of right ventricle (RV) from a pericardial effusion causing cardiac tamponade.

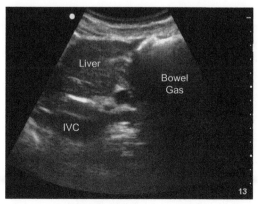

Fig. 19. Dilated inferior vena cava (IVC) from a pericardial effusion causing cardiac tamponade.

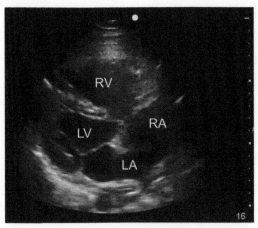

Fig. 20. Right ventricular (RV) dilation from a massive pulmonary embolism. RA, right atrium; RV, right ventricle; LA, left atrium; LV, left ventricle.

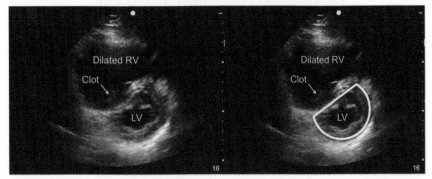

Fig. 21. Septal bowing into the LV, otherwise known as the D-sign, on parasternal short-axis view of the heart.

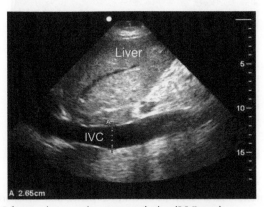

Fig. 22. Dilated IVC from a large pulmonary embolus (26.5 mm).

ventricular dilation. In this view, instead of its typical circular appearance, the left ventricle appears more like the letter D (see **Fig. 21**).

It is important to bear in mind that these sonographic findings must be taken in the context of the entire clinical picture, as many of these findings can also be seen with long-standing chronic obstructive pulmonary disease, obstructive sleep apnea, pulmonary hypertension, and right-sided myocardial infarction. Evaluation of the diameter of the right ventricular wall can help distinguish between acute and chronic right ventricular dilation and right ventricular dysfunction. Patients with chronic right ventricular strain will typically have a right ventricular wall thickness greater than 6 mm.[14] In addition, most patients with chronic right ventricular dysfunction will demonstrate global hypokinesis, whereas patients with a large, acute pulmonary embolism may exhibit hypokinesis of the right ventricular free wall and base, but normal contractility of the right ventricular apex. This apical sparing is known as the McConnell sign, and has been shown to have specificity of 94% and sensitivity of 77% for diagnosing an acute pulmonary embolism.[15]

These findings on the CORE scan in a hemodynamically unstable patient or in a patient in cardiac arrest should prompt the clinician to consider a large pulmonary embolism, and to contemplate initiation of thrombolytic therapy immediately.[16]

During the CORE scan, the heart should also be assessed to evaluate global contractility and estimate the ejection fraction. This information can be very useful in guiding fluid resuscitation and titrating doses of vasopressor agents.

To evaluate global function, obtain a parasternal long-axis view of the heart and examine the diameter of the left ventricle during systole and diastole. On global assessment, the heart's contractility can be generally categorized as either hyperdynamic, normal, mild to moderately decreased, or severely dysfunctional. To obtain a quantitative evaluation of the contractility of the left ventricle, use M-mode to evaluate the fractional shortening of the left ventricular diameter during systole and diastole. Fractional shortening can be calculated using the following formula:

Fractional shortening (%) = [(EDD − ESD)/EDD] × 100

where ESD is the end-systolic diameter measured between the ventricular walls just distal to the tips of the mitral valve leaflets, and EDD is the end-diastolic diameter measured between the ventricular walls at the same distance distal to the mitral valve leaflets (**Fig. 23**).

Studies have shown that a fractional shortening of 30% to 45% correlates with a normal ejection fraction.[17] Note that an M-mode tracing in a normal heart will show the left ventricular walls almost touching completely during systole with a high fractional shortening (**Fig. 24**).

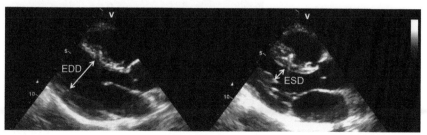

Fig. 23. End-diastolic diameter (EDD) and end-systolic diameter (ESD) on B-mode in a normal heart.

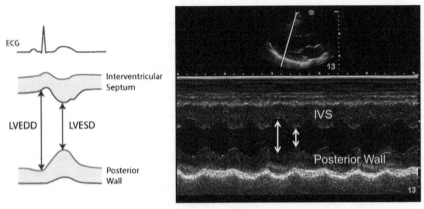

Fig. 24. Left ventricular end-diastolic diameter (LVEDD) and end-systolic diameter (LVESD) on M-mode in a normal heart. IVS, interventricular septum.

In a poorly contracting heart, the M-mode tracing demonstrates wide systolic separation between the ventricular walls and a low fractional shortening (**Fig. 25**). Remember that estimating fractional shortening is a quick and easy way to estimate systolic function at the bedside, and should be used in conjunction will the entire clinical picture.

Other ways to assess the ventricular contractility include assessing the E-point septal separation (EPSS). To evaluate the EPSS, obtain a parasternal long-axis view of the heart. With normal contractility, the anterior mitral leaflet should touch the septum during diastole. The distance separating the anterior mitral leaflet and the septum can be easily evaluated in M-mode (**Fig. 26**). With the cursor overlying the distal tip of the anterior mitral leaflet, assess the M-mode tracing for a characteristic pattern of two repeating waves. The taller first wave is the E-wave, which reflects the initial opening of the mitral valve to allow passive filling of the left ventricle. The smaller, second wave is the A-wave, which corresponds to left atrial contraction at the end of diastole.[18]

As cardiac contractility decreases, EPSS increases. Studies have shown that an EPSS greater than 1 cm correlates with a generally low ejection fraction (**Fig. 27**).[19] Of note, EPSS will not accurately predict ejection fraction in patients with mitral valve

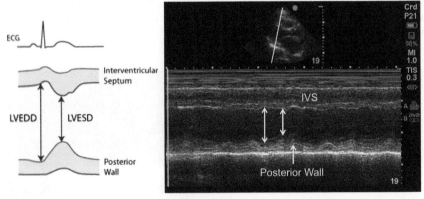

Fig. 25. LVEDD and LVESD on M-mode in a patient with a low ejection fraction and atrial fibrillation.

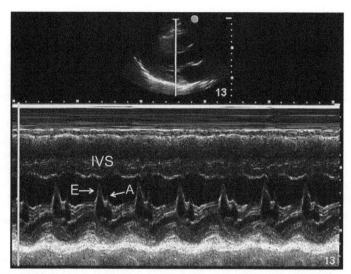

Fig. 26. Normal E-point septal separation (EPSS) where the anterior mitral valve touches the septum during diastole. A, left atrial contraction; E, initial opening of mitral valve; IVS, interventricular septum.

stenosis, mitral valve regurgitation, aortic regurgitation, or extreme left ventricular hypertrophy.

It is important to realize that there are other ultrasonographic methods available to evaluate cardiac contractility and ejection fraction. Many of these methods require specialized ultrasound software and are more time-intensive than the calculations commonly used in the CORE scan. Time and situation permitting, it is useful to learn and apply these calculations during patient management after interventions for acute resuscitation.

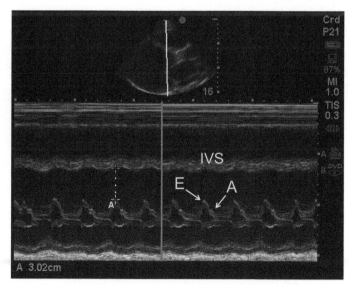

Fig. 27. Abnormally large EPSS from a patient with dilated cardiomyopathy and decreased ejection fraction.

BEDSIDE AORTA ULTRASONOGRAPHY

As part of the CORE scan, the abdominal aorta is evaluated for the presence of abnormalities that would require immediate intervention, such as an aortic aneurysm or aortic dissection. Using a low-frequency curvilinear transducer, obtain a transverse view of the IVC, aorta, and vertebral body just below the xiphoid process. Identifying all three structures in relation to each other will help prevent misidentification of any one of the structures during the scan (**Fig. 28**).

Once the aorta has been identified in this view, slide the probe toward the patient's left and center the aorta in the middle of the ultrasound screen. Scan through the abdominal aorta from the subxiphoid region down through the aortic bifurcation. The normal abdominal aorta diameter varies with age and gender. In general, the infrarenal aorta should measure less than 2.3 cm in males and less than 1.9 cm in females.[20] Evaluate the aorta for the presence of an aneurysm (>3.0 cm in diameter), focal dilation of the distal segment greater than 1.5 times the diameter of the proximal segment, lack of normal tapering distally, or the presence of any intraluminal thrombus (**Fig. 29**). Use gentle pressure and compression to help displace any bowel gas obstructing the view of the aorta, and obtain measurements of the aorta from outer wall to outer wall. If the aorta cannot be adequately visualized from the anterior approach, a longitudinal view of the aorta can be obtained using the liver as a window from the lateral approach (**Fig. 30**).

The aorta should also be evaluated for any sonographic signs of dissection. Note that most abdominal aortic dissections are usually an extension of a thoracic aortic dissection.[21] On ultrasonography, the presence of a hyperechoic intimal flap will be seen with an acute aortic dissection (**Fig. 31**).

If an abdominal aortic aneurysm or dissection is visualized, and the patient's clinical picture is concerning for sequelae from either of these conditions, resuscitation measures should be initiated immediately and the patient should undergo emergent intervention.

BEDSIDE IVC ULTRASONOGRAPHY

After the aorta has been evaluated, the IVC should be assessed to determine the status of the patient's intravascular volume. The absolute diameter of the IVC provides an estimation of the patient's central venous pressure.[22] Sonographic imaging of the IVC can be obtained via the anterior view (**Fig. 32**), or via the lateral view using the liver as an acoustic window (**Fig. 33**). It is important to obtain the best view of the IVC entering into the right atrium of the heart during the evaluation.

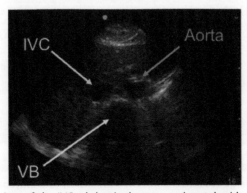

Fig. 28. Transverse view of the IVC, abdominal aorta, and vertebral body (VB).

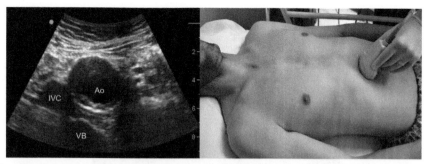

Fig. 29. Abdominal aortic aneurysm (4 cm in diameter) with intraluminal thrombus. Ao, aorta; IVC, inferior vena cava; VB, vertebral body.

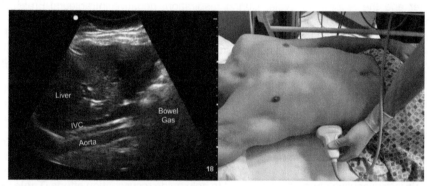

Fig. 30. Evaluation of abdominal aorta using the liver as a window from the lateral approach.

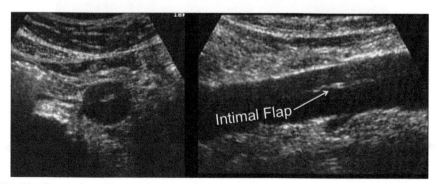

Fig. 31. Short-axis and long-axis views of an aortic dissection with hyperechoic intimal flap.

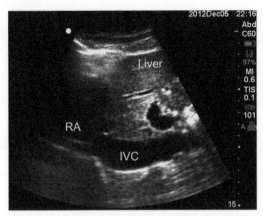

Fig. 32. Evaluation of the inferior vena cava (IVC) through the anterior approach.

The IVC is a highly compliant vessel, whose size varies with changes in total body water and the respiratory cycle. During respiration, negative intrapleural pressure develops, which results in increased venous return to the heart. As flow increases through the IVC, intraluminal pressure decreases and the diameter of the highly compliant IVC decreases. The difference in diameter at inspiration (IVC_i) and expiration (IVC_e) is referred to as the collapsibility index (also known as the caval index, CI) and is defined as:

$$\frac{IVCe - IVCi}{IVCe}$$

The CI has been shown to be higher in patients with shock, and can also be used to determine whether a patient has low central venous pressures. Recently, there has been increased interest in using the IVC diameter to help predict the extent of a patient's intravascular volume depletion and to help guide resuscitation efforts (**Table 2**).

It is important to remember that patients who are receiving positive pressure ventilation will have reversal of the IVC dynamics described here. Evaluating volume

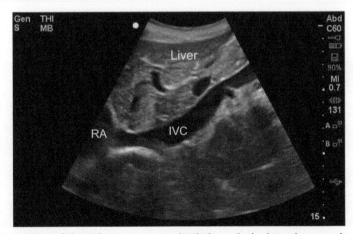

Fig. 33. Evaluation of the inferior vena cava (IVC) through the lateral approach.

Table 2
Correlation between IVC measurements and central venous pressure/right atrial pressure

IVC Diameter (mm)	% of Inspiratory Collapse	Estimated RA Pressure (cm H₂O)	Clinical Correlation
<15	100	0–5	Hypovolemic or distributive shock
15–25	>50	5–10	Shock
15–25	<50	11–15	Cardiogenic or obstructive shock
>25	<50	16–20	Cardiogenic or obstructive shock
>25	0	>20	Right-sided heart failure, massive PE, ARDS, pulmonary HTN, etc

Abbreviations: ARDS, acute respiratory distress syndrome; HTN, hypertension; IVC, inferior vena cava; PE, pulmonary embolism; RA, right atrium.

responsiveness with serial measurements of the IVC diameter can help guide resuscitation attempts.

According to recent literature, there are typically 3 common sites of measurement along the IVC (**Fig. 34**):

1. At the diaphragmatic junction (DJ)
2. Two centimeters distal to the hepatic vein inlet (2HVJ)
3. At the left renal vein junction (LRVJ).

Recent studies have suggested that measurements at 2HVJ provide the most consistent data over the course of the resuscitation attempts.

BEDSIDE EVALUATION FOR INTRAPERITONEAL FREE FLUID

Part of the CORE scan requires evaluation of the abdomen for the presence of intraperitoneal free fluid. The three main views that are recommended include evaluation of

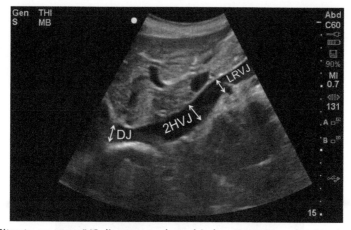

Fig. 34. Sites to measure IVC diameter and caval index. 2HVJ, 2 cm distal to hepatic vein inlet; DJ, diaphragmatic junction; LRVJ, left renal vein junction.

the right upper quadrant and the hepatorenal fossa, the left upper quadrant and the splenorenal fossa, and the suprapubic region to assess the retrovesicular space. In most situations, a quick assessment of the right upper quadrant should provide enough information to determine whether there is any intraperitoneal free fluid present. This portion of the body is the most dependent when a patient is lying supine. If the patient is sitting upright or if the head of the bed is elevated, the pelvis will be the most dependent portion where fluid will accumulate.

If the patient has intraperitoneal free fluid present, a dark anechoic stripe will be seen between the liver and the right kidney (**Fig. 35**), between the spleen and the left kidney (**Fig. 36**), or posterior to the bladder (**Fig. 37**).

In most circumstances, intraperitoneal free fluid accumulates as a result of trauma, although it can also be seen with rupture of an abdominal aortic aneurysm, rupture of an ectopic pregnancy, hemorrhage from an adnexal cyst or mass, spontaneous rupture or hemorrhage from a large hemangioma or neoplastic mass, or large viscus perforation. It is important to remember that it is difficult to distinguish between a small amount of ascites and intraperitoneal hemorrhage on bedside ultrasonography. Clinical correlation is required to determine the best approach to resuscitation if intraperitoneal hemorrhage is suspected based on the CORE scan. Serial scans are useful to determine whether the amount of intraperitoneal fluid is increasing during resuscitation attempts, and to help guide definitive intervention options.

BEDSIDE VASCULAR ULTRASONOGRAPHY

The final part of the CORE scan is to perform bedside ultrasonography to evaluate for the presence of deep venous thrombosis (DVT). The majority of hemodynamically significant pulmonary emboli arise from DVTs from the lower extremities.[23] The venous ultrasonography portion of the CORE scan focuses on the sites where most DVTs are likely to form: the common femoral vein, the proximal superficial femoral vein, and the popliteal vein.

On ultrasonography, veins will appear as oval-shaped hypoechoic structures running alongside round, thicker-walled arteries.[24] Color or pulse-wave Doppler can be used to distinguish veins from adjacent arteries (**Fig. 38**).

Normal veins should collapse completely when pressure is applied over them with the ultrasound transducer (**Fig. 39**). If the vein does not compress, there may be an

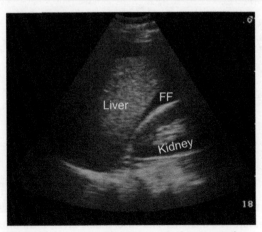

Fig. 35. Free fluid (FF) in the hepatorenal space or Morison's pouch.

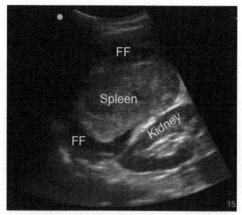

Fig. 36. Free fluid (FF) in the splenorenal space and around the spleen.

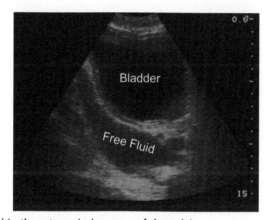

Fig. 37. Free fluid in the retrovesicular space of the pelvis.

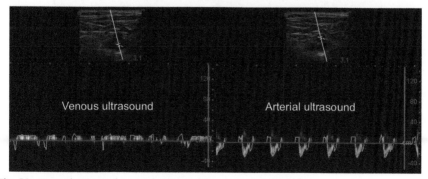

Fig. 38. Normal vein and normal artery with pulse-wave Doppler.

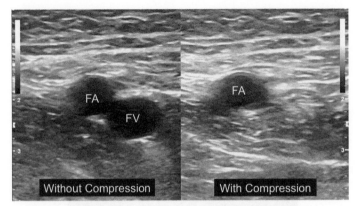

Fig. 39. Normal vein collapsing under transducer compression. FA, femoral artery; FV, femoral vein.

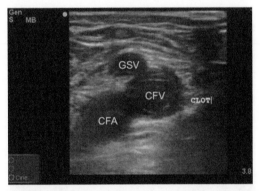

Fig. 40. Hyperechoic clot in the common femoral vein (CFV) and greater saphenous vein (GSV). CFA, common femoral artery.

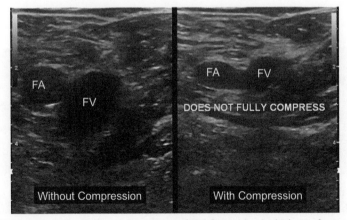

Fig. 41. Hyperechoic clot in the proximal superficial femoral vein (FV). FA, femoral artery.

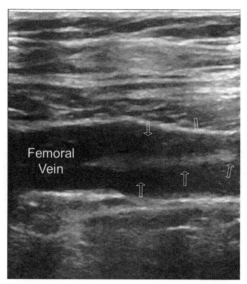

Fig. 42. Longitudinal view of a hyperechoic clot in the femoral vein (*arrows* indicate clot burden).

intraluminal clot preventing the edges from opposing one another.[25] Acute clots may not be easily visible on ultrasonography, as they are of the same echogenicity as the surrounding venous blood. As clot ages, it becomes more hyperechoic, and can be easily visualized in the lumen of the target vessel (**Fig. 40**).

Box 1
The CORE scan: concentrated overview of resuscitative efforts

1. Is the endotracheal tube in the trachea?
2. Are both lungs being ventilated?
3. Is there a tension pneumothorax that needs to be treated?
4. Is there a pleural effusion or hemothorax that needs to be addressed?
5. Does the patient still have cardiac activity?
6. Does the patient have a pericardial effusion and cardiac tamponade?
7. Is the right ventricle acutely dilated from a large pulmonary embolus?
8. Does the patient have the McConnell sign?
9. How is the heart contracting?
10. What is the estimated ejection fraction of the heart?
11. Does the patient have a symptomatic abdominal aortic aneurysm?
12. What is the intravascular volume status based on evaluation of the inferior vena cava?
13. Is the patient's inferior vena cava responding to intravascular volume replacement?
14. Does the patient have intraperitoneal free fluid?
15. Does the patient have a deep venous thrombosis?

Using ultrasonography, the common femoral vein, proximal superficial femoral vein, and popliteal veins can be evaluated rapidly to determine whether an intraluminal clot is present (**Fig. 41**). Once an intraluminal clot has been visualized, a longitudinal view of the affected vessel can be assessed to determine the extent of the clot (**Fig. 42**).

If a DVT is visualized during the CORE scan, appropriate anticoagulation should be initiated immediately, and the possibility of a large, downstream, pulmonary embolism should be considered as the cause of the patient's hemodynamic compromise.

SUMMARY

The CORE scan should be used during the evaluation and assessment of patients who present with acute, undifferentiated clinical decompensation. The targeted sonographic views of the CORE scan can be used to diagnose potentially reversible causes of cardiopulmonary and vascular compromise. During the CORE scan, the overall clinical picture will determine the order in which the individual scans are performed. When used in conjunction with clinical findings, the CORE scan can improve diagnostic accuracy and can help guide resuscitative efforts (**Box 1**).

REFERENCES

1. Scalea TM, Rodriguez A, Chiu WC, et al. Focused assessment with sonography for trauma (FAST): results from an international consensus conference. J Trauma 1999;46(3):466–72.
2. Kirkpatrick AW, Sirois M, Laupland KB, et al. Hand-held thoracic sonography for detecting post-traumatic pneumothoraces: the extended focused assessment with sonography for trauma (EFAST). J Trauma 2004;57:288–95.
3. Atkinson RT, McAuley DJ, Kendall RJ, et al. Abdominal and cardiac evaluation with sonography in shock (ACES): an approach by emergency physicians for the use of ultrasound in patients with undifferentiated hypotension. Emerg Med J 2009;26(2):87–91.
4. Lanctot YF, Valois M, Bealieu Y. EGLS: echo guided life support. An algorithmic approach to undifferentiated shock. Crit Ultrasound J 2011;3:129.
5. Lichtenstein DA, Karakitsos D. Integrating ultrasound in the hemodynamic evaluation of acute circulatory failure (FALLS—the fluid administration limited by lung sonography protocol). J Crit Care 2012;27(5):533.e11–9.
6. Seif D, Perera P, Mailhot T, et al. Bedside ultrasound in resuscitation and the rapid ultrasound in shock protocol. Crit Care Res Pract 2012;2012:503254.
7. Werner SL, Smith CE, Goldstein JR, et al. Pilot study to evaluate the accuracy of ultrasonography in confirming endotracheal tube placement. Ann Emerg Med 2007;49:75–80.
8. Lichtenstein DA, Meziere G, Lascols N, et al. Ultrasound diagnosis of occult pneumothorax. Crit Care Med 2005;33:1231–8.
9. Lichtenstein D, Meziere G, Biderman P, et al. The "lung point": an ultrasound sign specific to pneumothorax. Intensive Care Med 2000;26(10):1434–40.
10. Goodman A, Perera P, Mailhot T, et al. The role of bedside ultrasound in the diagnosis of pericardial effusion and cardiac tamponade. J Emerg Trauma Shock 2012;5(1):72–5.
11. Wann S, Passen E. Echocardiography in pericardial disease. J Am Soc Echocardiogr 2008;21(1):7–13.
12. Tirado A, Wu T, Noble VE, et al. Ultrasound-guided procedures in the emergency department—diagnostic and therapeutic asset. Emerg Med Clin North Am 2013; 31(1):117–49.

13. Borloz MP, Frohna WJ, Phillips CA, et al. Emergency department focused bedside echocardiography in massive pulmonary embolism. J Emerg Med 2011;41(6):658–60.
14. Wood KE. Major pulmonary embolism: review of a pathophysiologic approach to the golden hour of hemodynamically significant pulmonary embolism. Chest 2002;121:877–905.
15. McConnell MV, Solomon SD, Rayan ME, et al. Regional right ventricular dysfunction detected by echocardiography in acute pulmonary embolism. Am J Cardiol 1996;78:469–73.
16. Labovitz AJ, Bierig M, Goldstein SA, et al. Focused cardiac ultrasound in the emergent setting: a consensus statement of the American Society of Echocardiography and the American College of Emergency Physicians. 2010. Available at: http://www.acep.org/. Accessed February, 2013.
17. Randazzo MR, Snoey ER, Levitt MA, et al. Accuracy of emergency physician assessment of left ventricular ejection fraction and central venous pressure using echocardiography. Acad Emerg Med 2003;10(9):973–7.
18. Perera P, Mailhot T, Riley D, et al. The RUSH exam: rapid Ultrasound in SHock in the evaluation of the critically ill. Emerg Med Clin North Am 2010;28(1):29–56.
19. Silverstein JR, Laffely NH, Rifkin RD. Quantitative estimation of left ventricular ejection fraction from mitral valve E-point to septal separation and comparison to magnetic resonance imaging. Am J Cardiol 2006;97(1):137–40.
20. Pedersen OM, Aslaksen A, Vik-Mo H. Ultrasound measurement of the luminal diameter of the abdominal aorta and iliac arteries in patients without vascular disease. J Vasc Surg 1993;17:596–601.
21. Bhatt S, Ghazale H, Dogra VS. Sonographic evaluation of the abdominal aorta. Ultrasound Clin 2007;2:437–53.
22. Jardin F, Vieillard-Baron A. Ultrasonographic examination of the venae cavae. Intensive Care Med 2006;32(2):203–6.
23. Poppiti R, Papinocolau G, Perese S. Limited B-mode venous scanning versus complete color flow duplex venous scanning for detection of proximal deep venous thrombosis. J Vasc Surg 1995;22:553–7.
24. Kline JA, O'Malley PM, Tayal VS, et al. Emergency clinician-performed compression ultrasonography for deep venous thrombosis of the lower extremity. Ann Emerg Med 2008;52(4):437–45.
25. Crisp JG, Lovato LM, Jang TB. Compression ultrasonography of the lower extremity with portable vascular ultrasonography can accurately detect deep venous thrombosis in the emergency department. Ann Emerg Med 2010;56(6):601–10.

Index

Note: Page numbers of article titles are in **boldface** type.

Crit Care Clin 30 (2014) 177–184
http://dx.doi.org/10.1016/S0749-0704(13)00106-1
0749-0704/14/$ – see front matter © 2014 Elsevier Inc. All rights reserved.

criticalcare.theclinics.com

Moving?

Make sure your subscription moves with you!

To notify us of your new address, find your **Clinics Account Number** (located on your mailing label above your name), and contact customer service at:

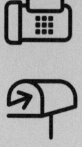

Email: journalscustomerservice-usa@elsevier.com

800-654-2452 (subscribers in the U.S. & Canada)
314-447-8871 (subscribers outside of the U.S. & Canada)

Fax number: 314-447-8029

**Elsevier Health Sciences Division
Subscription Customer Service
3251 Riverport Lane
Maryland Heights, MO 63043**

*To ensure uninterrupted delivery of your subscription, please notify us at least 4 weeks in advance of move.

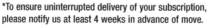

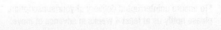